T0229313

Contraception

Editors

PAMELA S. LOTKE
BLISS KANESHIRO

OBSTETRICS AND GYNECOLOGY CLINICS OF NORTH AMERICA

www.obgyn.theclinics.com

Consulting Editor
WILLIAM F. RAYBURN

December 2015 • Volume 42 • Number 4

ELSEVIER

1600 John F. Kennedy Boulevard • Suite 1800 • Philadelphia, Pennsylvania, 19103-2899

http://www.theclinics.com

OBSTETRICS AND GYNECOLOGY CLINICS OF NORTH AMERICA Volume 42, Number 4
December 2015 ISSN 0889-8545, ISBN-13: 978-0-323-40258-3

Editor: Kerry Holland
Developmental Editor: Kristen Helm

Obstetrics and Gynecology Clinics (ISSN 0889-8545) is published quarterly by Elsevier Inc., 360 Park Avenue South, New York, NY 10010-1710. Months of issue are March, June, September, and December. Periodicals postage paid at New York, NY, and additional mailing offices. Subscription price per year is $310.00 (US individuals), $545.00 (US institutions), $155.00 (US students), $370.00 (Canadian individuals), $688.00 (Canadian institutions), $225.00 (Canadian students), $450.00 (international individuals), $688.00 (international institutions), and $225.00 (international students). To receive student/resident rate, orders must be accompanied by name of affiliated institution, date of term, and the signature of program/residency coordinator on institution letterhead. Orders will be billed at individual rate until proof of status is received. Foreign air speed delivery is included in all *Clinics* subscription prices. All prices are subject to change without notice. POSTMASTER: Send address changes to *Obstetrics and Gynecology Clinics*, Elsevier Health Sciences Division, Subscription Customer Service, 3251 Riverport Lane, Maryland Heights, MO 63043. **Customer Service: Telephone: 1-800-654-2452 (U.S. and Canada); 314-447-8871 (outside U.S. and Canada). Fax: 314-447-8029. E-mail: journalscustomerservice-usa@elsevier.com (for print support); journalsonlinesupport-usa@elsevier. com (for online support).**

Reprints. For copies of 100 or more of articles in this publication, please contact the Commercial Reprints Department, Elsevier Inc., 360 Park Avenue South, New York, New York 10010-1710. Tel.: 212-633-3874; Fax: 212-633-3820; E-mail: reprints@elsevier.com.

Obstetrics and Gynecology Clinics of North America is also published in Spanish by McGraw-Hill Interamericana Editores S.A., P.O. Box 5-237, 06500, Mexico; in Portuguese by Reichmann and Affonso Editores, Rio de Janeiro, Brazil; and in Greek by Paschalidis Medical Publications, Athens, Greece.

Obstetrics and Gynecology Clinics of North America is covered in MEDLINE/PubMed (Index Medicus), Excerpta Medica, Current Concepts/Clinical Medicine, Science Citation Index, BIOSIS, CINAHL, and ISI/BIOMED.

Contributors

CONSULTING EDITOR

WILLIAM F. RAYBURN, MD, MBA
Associate Dean, Continuing Medical Education and Professional Development, Distinguished Professor and Emeritus Chair, Obstetrics and Gynecology, University of New Mexico School of Medicine, Albuquerque, New Mexico

EDITORS

PAMELA S. LOTKE, MD, MPH
Director, Division of Family Planning and Preventive Care, Department of Obstetrics and Gynecology, MedStar Washington Hospital Center, Washington, DC

BLISS KANESHIRO, MD, MPH
Associate Professor, Director of the Family Planning Fellowship and the Division of Family Planning, Department of Obstetrics, Gynecology, and Women's Health, Kapiolani Medical Center for Women and Children, University of Hawaii John A. Burns School of Medicine, Honolulu, Hawaii

AUTHORS

PAULA H. BEDNAREK, MD, MPH
Associate Professor, Department of Obstetrics and Gynecology, Oregon Health and Science University, Portland, Oregon

LYNDSEY S. BENSON, MD, MS
Fellow in Family Planning, Department of Obstetrics and Gynecology, University of Washington, Seattle, Washington

HOLLY BULLOCK, MD, MPH
Department of Obstetrics, Gynecology, and Women's Health, University of Hawaii John A. Burns School of Medicine, Honolulu, Hawaii

ALISON EDELMAN, MD, MPH
Professor, Department of Obstetrics and Gynecology, Oregon Health and Science University, Portland, Oregon

EMMAKATE FRIEDLANDER, MD
Family Planning Fellow, Department of Obstetrics, Gynecology and Women's Health, University of Hawaii John A. Burns School of Medicine, Honolulu, Hawaii

DANIEL GROSSMAN, MD
Vice President for Research, Ibis Reproductive Health, Oakland, California; Professor, Department of Obstetrics, Gynecology and Reproductive Sciences, Bixby Center for Global Reproductive Health, University of California, San Francisco, San Francisco, California

LEO HAN, MD
Instructor, Department of Obstetrics and Gynecology, Oregon Health and Science University, Portland, Oregon

MICHELLE M. ISLEY, MD, MPH
Assistant Professor, Department of Obstetrics and Gynecology, Ohio State University, Columbus, Ohio

JEFFREY T. JENSEN, MD, MPH
Professor, Department of Obstetrics and Gynecology, Oregon Health and Science University, Portland, Oregon

BLISS KANESHIRO, MD, MPH
Associate Professor, Director of the Family Planning Fellowship and the Division of Family Planning, Department of Obstetrics, Gynecology, and Women's Health, Kapiolani Medical Center for Women and Children, University of Hawaii John A. Burns School of Medicine, Honolulu, Hawaii

PAMELA S. LOTKE, MD, MPH
Director, Division of Family Planning and Preventive Care, Department of Obstetrics and Gynecology, MedStar Washington Hospital Center, Washington, DC

ERIN E. McCOY, MPH
Program and Research Manager, Department of Obstetrics and Gynecology, University of Washington, Seattle, Washington

ELIZABETH A. MICKS, MD, MPH
Assistant Professor, Department of Obstetrics and Gynecology, University of Washington, Seattle, Washington

CHAILEE MOSS, MD
Clinical Instructor, Department of Obstetrics and Gynecology, Ohio State University, Columbus, Ohio

EVA PATIL, MD
Fellow in Family Planning, Department of Obstetrics and Gynecology, Oregon Health and Science University, Portland, Oregon

SARAH W. PRAGER, MD, MAS
Associate Professor, Department of Obstetrics and Gynecology, University of Washington, Seattle, Washington

SHANDHINI RAIDOO, MD
Fellow in Family Planning, Department of Obstetrics, Gynecology, and Women's Health, Kapiolani Medical Center for Women and Children, University of Hawaii John A. Burns School of Medicine, Honolulu, Hawaii

JENNIFER SALCEDO, MD, MPH, MPP
Department of Obstetrics, Gynecology, and Women's Health, University of Hawaii John A. Burns School of Medicine, Honolulu, Hawaii

RENI SOON, MD, MPH
Assistant Professor, Department of Obstetrics, Gynecology, and Women's Health, University of Hawaii John A. Burns School of Medicine, Honolulu, Hawaii

MARY TSCHANN, MPH
Junior Researcher, Department of Obstetrics, Gynecology, and Women's Health, University of Hawaii John A. Burns School of Medicine, Honolulu, Hawaii

WAN-JU WU, MD, MPH
Resident Physician, Department of Obstetrics and Gynecology, Oregon Health and Science University, Portland, Oregon

Contents

Foreword: Contraceptive Needs—A Gateway to the Obstetrician-Gynecologist's Office xiii

William F. Rayburn

Preface: Contraception xv

Pamela S. Lotke and Bliss Kaneshiro

Increasing Use of Long-Acting Reversible Contraception to Decrease Unplanned Pregnancy 557

Pamela S. Lotke

Unintended pregnancy remains high in the United States, accounting for one-half of pregnancies. Both contraceptive nonuse and imperfect use contribute to unplanned pregnancies. Long-acting reversible contraception (LARC) have greater efficacy than shorter acting methods. Data from large studies show that unplanned pregnancy rates are lower among women using LARC. However, overall use of LARC is low; of the reproductive age women using contraception, less than 10% are LARC users. Barriers include lack of knowledge and high up-front cost, and prevent more widespread use. Overcoming these barriers and increasing the number of women using LARC will decrease unplanned pregnancies and abortions.

Immediate Postpartum Intrauterine Contraception Insertion 569

Sarah W. Prager and Erin E. McCoy

The immediate postpartum period is a favorable time for initiating contraception because women who have recently given birth are often highly motivated to use contraception, pregnancy is excluded, and the hospital setting offers convenience for patients and providers. This article addresses immediate postpartum intrauterine contraception (IUC) insertion for copper and levonorgestrel IUC. Immediate postpartum IUC is safe and effective, with a majority of IUC devices retained at 6 and 12 months. There are increased rates of expulsion, compared with delayed postpartum insertion and interval insertion, which need to be weighed against the risk of patients not returning for postpartum follow-up.

Immediate Intrauterine Device Insertion Following Surgical Abortion 583

Eva Patil and Paula H. Bednarek

Placement of an intrauterine device (IUD) immediately after a first or second trimester surgical abortion is safe and convenient and decreases the risk of repeat unintended pregnancy. Immediate postabortion IUD placement is not recommended in the setting of postprocedure hemorrhage, uterine perforation, infection, or hematometra. Otherwise, there are few contraindications to IUD placement following surgical abortion. Sexually transmitted infection screening should follow US Centers for Disease Control and

Prevention guidelines. No additional antibiotics are needed beyond those used for the abortion. Placing immediate postabortion IUDs makes highly-effective long-acting reversible contraception more accessible to women.

Therapeutic Options for Unscheduled Bleeding Associated with Long-Acting Reversible Contraception   593

EmmaKate Friedlander and Bliss Kaneshiro

Long-acting reversible contraception (LARC) is the most effective form of reversible contraception. Although most women are satisfied with LARC methods, unscheduled bleeding and spotting are common reasons for method dissatisfaction and discontinuation. This systematic analysis of the current literature delineates treatment options for unscheduled bleeding related to LARC use. Although consistent results are lacking, all devices seem to have the best response to nonsteroidal antiinflammatory drugs for 5 to 7 days or the antifibrinolytic agent tranexamic acid. Additional studies are necessary to identify improved treatment interventions for unscheduled bleeding with LARC use.

Contraceptive Coverage and the Affordable Care Act   605

Mary Tschann and Reni Soon

A major goal of the Patient Protection and Affordable Care Act is reducing healthcare spending by shifting the focus of healthcare toward preventive care. Preventive services, including all FDA-approved contraception, must be provided to patients without cost-sharing under the ACA. No-cost contraception has been shown to increase uptake of highly effective birth control methods and reduce unintended pregnancy and abortion; however, some institutions and corporations argue that providing contraceptive coverage infringes on their religious beliefs. The contraceptive coverage mandate is evolving due to legal challenges, but it has already demonstrated success in reducing costs and improving access to contraception.

Over-the-Counter Access to Oral Contraceptives   619

Daniel Grossman

Making oral contraceptives (OCs) available over the counter (OTC) could help to reduce the high rate of unintended pregnancy in the United States. Surveys show widespread support for OTC access to OCs among US women. Studies indicate that women can accurately use checklists to identify contraindications to OCs. Continuation is as good or better among OTC users compared with women using OCs obtained by prescription. Women and clinicians have expressed concerns related to making OCs available OTC. These concerns can be addressed by existing data or through research required by the Food and Drug Administration as part of the application to make OCs available OTC.

Providing Contraception to Adolescents   631

Shandhini Raidoo and Bliss Kaneshiro

Adolescents have high rates of unintended pregnancy and face unique reproductive health challenges. Providing confidential contraceptive services to adolescents is important in reducing the rate of unintended pregnancy. Long-acting contraception such as the intrauterine device and contraceptive implant are recommended as first-line contraceptives for adolescents because they are highly effective with few side effects. The use of barrier methods to prevent sexually transmitted infections should be encouraged. Adolescents have limited knowledge of reproductive health and contraceptive options, and their sources of information are often unreliable. Access to contraception is available through a variety of resources that continue to expand.

Safety and Efficacy of Contraceptive Methods for Obese and Overweight Women   **647**

Pamela S. Lotke and Bliss Kaneshiro

Increasing rates of obesity have become a major public health challenge. Given the added health risks that obese women have during pregnancy, preventing unwanted pregnancy is imperative. Clinicians who provide contraception must understand the efficacy, risks, and the weight changes associated with various contraceptive methods. Despite differences in the pharmacokinetics and pharmacodynamics of hormonal contraceptives in overweight and obese women, efficacy does not appear to be severely impacted. Both estrogen-containing contraceptives and obesity increase the risk of venous thromboembolism, but the absolute risk remains acceptably low in reproductive age women.

Contraceptive Method Initiation: Using the Centers for Disease Control and Prevention Selected Practice Guidelines   **659**

Wan-Ju Wu and Alison Edelman

The US Selected Practice Recommendations is a companion document to the Medical Eligibility Criteria for Contraceptive Use that focuses on how providers can use contraceptive methods most effectively as well as problem-solve common issues that may arise. These guidelines serve to help clinicians provide contraception safely as well as to decrease barriers that prevent or delay a woman from obtaining a desired method. This article summarizes the Selected Practice Recommendations on timing of contraceptive initiation, examinations, and tests needed prior to starting a method and any necessary follow-up.

Why Stop Now? Extended and Continuous Regimens of Combined Hormonal Contraceptive Methods   **669**

Lyndsey S. Benson and Elizabeth A. Micks

Combined hormonal contraceptives (CHCs) have traditionally been prescribed in 28-day cycles, with 21 days of active hormones followed by a 7-day hormone-free interval. Extended and continuous CHC regimens, defined as regimens with greater than 28 days of active hormones, offer many benefits, including a decrease in estrogen-withdrawal symptoms and likely greater efficacy because of more reliable ovulation suppression. Bleeding profiles are favorable, and unscheduled bleeding decreases over time with these regimens. Extended and continuous regimens of combined oral contraceptives and the contraceptive vaginal ring are safe and have high user acceptability and satisfaction. However, despite numerous benefits, extended and continuous CHC regimens are underused.

Does the Progestogen Used in Combined Hormonal Contraception Affect Venous
Thrombosis Risk?   683

Leo Han and Jeffrey T. Jensen

Combined hormonal contraceptives (CHCs) use a combination of estrogen and progestogen to provide contraception. The most important risk of using CHCs is venous thromboembolism (VTE). It is unclear whether the type of progestogen used in a method augments that risk. Although the evidence supporting an increase in thrombosis risk is not conclusive, neither is the evidence supporting the benefit of newer progestogens in terms of tolerability or continuation. The benefits of CHCs outweigh the risks and the absolute risk of VTE remains small. A balanced discussion of potential risks and benefits of particular CHC formulations is warranted during contraception counseling.

Emergency Contraception: Do Your Patients Have a Plan B?   699

Holly Bullock and Jennifer Salcedo

Emergency contraception is used after unprotected sex, inadequately protected sex, or sexual assault to reduce the risk of pregnancy. Of emergency contraceptive methods available in the United States, the copper intrauterine device has the highest efficacy, followed by ulipristal acetate, levonorgestrel-containing emergency contraceptive pills, and the Yuzpe method. However, access to the most effective methods is limited. Although advanced prescription of emergency contraceptive pills and counseling on emergency contraception to all reproductive-aged women is recommended, women should be advised to contact their health care providers after taking emergency contraceptive pills to discuss possible copper intrauterine device placement and other follow-up.

Sterilization: A Review and Update   713

Chailee Moss and Michelle M. Isley

Sterilization is a frequently used method of contraception. Female sterilization is performed 3 times more frequently than male sterilization, and it can be performed immediately postpartum or as an interval procedure. Methods include mechanical occlusion, coagulation, or tubal excision. Female sterilization can be performed using an abdominal approach, or via laparoscopy or hysteroscopy. When an abdominal approach or laparoscopy is used, sterilization occurs immediately. When hysteroscopy is used, tubal occlusion occurs over time, and additional testing is needed to confirm tubal occlusion. Comprehensive counseling about sterilization should include discussion about male sterilization (vasectomy) and long-acting reversible contraceptive methods.

Index   725

OBSTETRICS AND GYNECOLOGY CLINICS

FORTHCOMING ISSUES

March 2016
**Management and Advanced Surgery
for Pelvic Floor Dysfunction**
Cheryl B. Iglesia, *Editor*

June 2016
Primary Care of Adult Women
James N. Woodruff and
Anita K. Blanchard, *Editors*

September 2016
Hysterectomy and the Alternatives
John A. Occhino and
Emanuel C. Trabuco, *Editors*

RECENT ISSUES

September 2015
**Obstetric and Gynecologic Hospitalists and
Laborists**
Brigid McCue and Jennifer A.
Tessmer-Tuck, *Editors*

June 2015
Best Practices in High-Risk Pregnancy
Lynn L. Simpson, *Editor*

March 2015
Reproductive Endocrinology
Michelle L. Matthews, *Editor*

ISSUE OF RELATED INTEREST

Medical Clinics of North America, May 2015 (Vol. 99, No. 3)
Women's Health
Joyce E. Wipf, *Editor*

THE CLINICS ARE AVAILABLE ONLINE!
Access your subscription at:
www.theclinics.com

Foreword

Contraceptive Needs— A Gateway to the Obstetrician- Gynecologist's Office

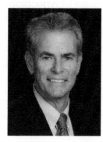

William F. Rayburn, MD, MBA
Consulting Editor

This issue of *Obstetrics and Gynecology Clinics of North America*, edited by Dr Pamela Lotke and Dr Bliss Kaneshiro, identifies the best topics for discussion about contraception. Most reproductive-aged women will seek out contraceptive care, which often serves as a gateway to the obstetrician-gynecologist office. Despite the fact that two-thirds to three-quarters of reproductive-age women use some form of contraception in the United States, approximately half of all pregnancies (6.7 million annually) are unintended. Therefore, an update about the spectrum of contraception methods is essential to readers of the *Obstetrics and Gynecology Clinics of North America*.

The editors have compiled an excellent list of topics worthy of our attention and sought the expertise of competent authors specializing in family planning. Multiple methods of contraception are highlighted in this issue, ranging from intrauterine contraception immediately postpartum or following surgical abortion, to emergency contraception, and sterilization. Our patients should be encouraged to choose a method from the most effective options while considering adverse events, length of use, and noncontraceptive benefits.

Throughout the issue, the authors encourage the reader to consider the following topics: when to begin contraception, how to manage women with medical issues (such as venous thrombosis risk), and return to fertility after discontinuation. The importance of counseling and strategies to enhance compliance are emphasized. The issue nicely addresses pertinent questions relating to age (especially adolescence), obesity, need for a Plan B, and when to discontinue contraception (or why stop?).

Current topics of particular interest to the reader deal with over-the-counter access to oral contraceptives, new guidelines from the Centers for Disease Control and Prevention (CDC), and contraceptive coverage and costs under the Affordable Care Act

Obstet Gynecol Clin N Am 42 (2015) xiii–xiv
http://dx.doi.org/10.1016/j.ogc.2015.08.006
0889-8545/15/$ – see front matter © 2015 Published by Elsevier Inc.

obgyn.theclinics.com

mandate. Many absolute and relative contraindications to hormonal contraception, according to the CDC, are described in detail. Basics for patient education in plain language are also emphasized. Emergency contraception for those using barrier contraception and short-acting hormonal methods should be part of that discussion.

I appreciate this contemporary overview compiled by Dr Lotke and Dr Kaneshiro. Strategies presented in this issue are especially relevant. While breast and pelvic exams and screening for sexually transmitted diseases and cervical cancer are important, most groups, including the American College of Obstetricians and Gynecologists, World Health Organization, and Royal College of Obstetricians and Gynecologists, agree that these procedures are not necessary before beginning or reinitiating a method of contraception. Furthermore, I anticipate that contraceptive technology will advance in the ensuing decade with fewer adverse events and improved compliance. We look forward to a timely update in another 5 years about the best contraceptive methods that provide our patients with high levels of satisfaction and continuation.

William F. Rayburn, MD, MBA
Continuing Medical Education &
Professional Development
MSC10 5580
1 University of New Mexico
Albuquerque, NM 87131-0001, USA

E-mail address:
wrayburn@salud.unm.edu

Preface

Contraception

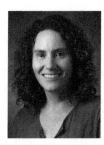 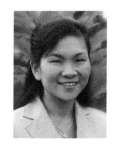

Pamela S. Lotke, MD, MPH   Bliss Kaneshiro, MD, MPH
Editors

We are thrilled to devote an issue to contraception at this junction in women's health care. The high rate of unplanned pregnancy that has plagued the United States for decades has started to decline in selected regions. As many are well aware, one-half of pregnancies in the country are unplanned, and 40% of unplanned pregnancies end in abortion. These statistics have remained stable for years. It represents a failure to empower women with the basic right to decide for themselves *if* and *when* to have children.

Several factors have empowered certain groups of women to make health decisions that are consistent with their reproductive life plan. These factors include access to evidence-based reproductive health education and the availability of effective contraception through either the Affordable Care Act's Contraceptive Mandate or local measures to increase access to contraception. In groups of women with education and access to effective contraceptive methods, we see marked declines in the rate of unintended pregnancy and abortion.

Intrauterine devices and contraceptive implants are key components of this progress. These methods of long-acting reversible contraception are safe and require little of the user to achieve perfect-use efficacy rates. It is crucial to ensure women have access to these methods, both financially and logistically. Understanding not just *who* are eligible candidates for these methods, but also *when* they can be initiated, is important to allow more women to take advantage of them.

The political, legal, and medical climates in this country affect women's reproductive options. To elucidate these connections, we have included discussions about the Affordable Care Act and the possibility of over-the-counter access to contraception. Certain vulnerable populations require special attention, and consideration of the specific concerns of adolescents and obese women is addressed. In addition, the family planning experts contributing to this issue provide in-depth information on best practice regarding use of combined hormonal contraception and sterilization, which remain the most commonly used methods of contraception.

Obstet Gynecol Clin N Am 42 (2015) xv–xvi
http://dx.doi.org/10.1016/j.ogc.2015.08.005
0889-8545/15/$ – see front matter © 2015 Published by Elsevier Inc.

obgyn.theclinics.com

Our goal is to provide readers with up-to-date information on how best to use the spectrum of contraceptive methods across a diverse patient population with respect to patient needs and safety. Ultimately, the best contraceptive method is one that a woman herself feels comfortable with and wants to continue. We aim to empower women and providers to find that method together.

Pamela S. Lotke, MD, MPH
Division of Family Planning
and Preventive Care
Department of Obstetrics
and Gynecology
MedStar Washington Hospital Center
106 Irving Street, NW
POB Suite 4700 North
Washington, DC 20010, USA

Bliss Kaneshiro, MD, MPH
Division of Family Planning
Department of Obstetrics and Gynecology
University of Hawaii
John A. Burns School of Medicine
1319 Punahou Street, #824
Honolulu, HI 96826, USA

E-mail addresses:
pamela.lotke@medstar.net (P.S. Lotke)
blissk@hawaii.edu (B. Kaneshiro)

Increasing Use of Long-Acting Reversible Contraception to Decrease Unplanned Pregnancy

 CrossMark

Pamela S. Lotke, MD, MPH

KEYWORDS

- Long-acting reversible contraception • Unintended pregnancy • Contraception
- Contraception counseling • Family planning

KEY POINTS

- Unintended pregnancy rates remain high in the United States, accounting for one-half of pregnancies.
- Women using short-acting contraception are 21 times more likely than women using long-acting reversible contraceptives (LARC) to have an unplanned pregnancy.
- Adolescents under 21 years old are twice as likely to have an unplanned pregnancy using short-acting methods than women 21 and over.
- Barriers include lack of knowledge and excess cost at the level of the woman, health care provider, and health care system.
- Overcoming these barriers and increasing the number of women using LARC will help to decrease unplanned pregnancies.

INTRODUCTION

Despite modern contraceptive methods, the unplanned pregnancy rate in the United States remains persistently high. The decline in the unplanned pregnancy rates from the 1980s and 1990s stalled by the turn of the century, and even worsened slightly between 2001 and 2006. Rates of unintended pregnancy are differentially distributed based on demographic factors. Just more than 10% of women 18 to 24 years of age experience an unplanned pregnancy each year, which is double the average for all women. Black women experience twice the rate of unplanned pregnancies as white women, and women with incomes below 100% of the federal poverty level have

Disclosures: Dr P. Lotke serves on an international advisory board for Bayer Healthcare and as a clinical trainer for Nexplanon (Merck).
Division of Family Planning and Preventive Care, Department of Obstetrics and Gynecology, MedStar Washington Hospital Center, 110 Irving Street, Northwest, Washington, DC 20010, USA
E-mail address: Pamela.lotke@medstar.net

Obstet Gynecol Clin N Am 42 (2015) 557–567
http://dx.doi.org/10.1016/j.ogc.2015.07.008
0889-8545/15/$ – see front matter © 2015 Elsevier Inc. All rights reserved.

5 times the rate of unplanned pregnancies as women with incomes at or above 200% of the poverty level.[1]

In the past few years, we have reason for optimism. A steady increase in the number of women using long-acting reversible contraception (LARC) including the contraceptive implant and intrauterine devices (IUD) has been noted. From 2002 to 2009, LARC use among reproductive age women more than tripled, from 2.4% to 8.5%.[2] Because LARC requires no effort after insertion to remain highly effective, efficacy with "typical" use approaches that of "perfect use."[3] The contraceptive failure risk is 20 times greater in women using short-acting methods than in women using LARC.[4] Greater efficacy, as well as higher continuation rates and satisfaction with LARC compared with other methods,[5–8] have resulted in decreased rates of unintended pregnancy among LARC users.[4,9–12]

EFFICACY OF LONG-ACTING REVERSIBLE CONTRACEPTION VERSUS SHORT-ACTING METHODS

A sizable body of evidence demonstrates greater efficacy of LARC than other methods of contraception. Most of this benefit comes from the difference between "typical" versus "perfect" use. Trussell[3] compared data from the literature on contraceptive efficacy in the research setting (perfect use) to estimates of efficacy from the National Survey of Family Growth in 1995 and 2002 (typical use). In these surveys, women self-reported their contraceptive method as well as lapses in use. Women who use condoms occasionally but not always are counted among condom users, and active pills users are counted together with women whose prescriptions have lapsed or have not picked up refills for some time.[3] Based on these "real-world" scenarios, the failure rate was 9% for the pill, patch, or ring. This is significantly higher than the 0.3% failure rates with perfect use reported in studies, and also higher than the typical failure rates with LARC (**Table 1**).[3] Other data on failure rates emerge from women seeking

Method	Typical Use (% Pregnant in First Year of Use)	Perfect Use (% Pregnant in First Year of Use)	Continuation at 1 y
Table 1 Contraceptive method failure and continuation after first year of use			
No method	85	85	—
Withdrawal	22	4	46
Male condom	18	2	43
Combined pills and progestin only pill	9	0.3	67
Evra patch	9	0.3	67
NuvaRing	9	0.3	67
Depo-Provera	6	0.2	56
ParaGard IUD	0.8	0.6	78
Mirena (LNG) IUD	0.2	0.2	80
Implanon	0.05	0.05	84
Female sterilization	0.5	0.5	100
Male sterilization	0.15	0.10	100

Abbreviation: IUD, intrauterine device.

Data from Trussell J. Contraceptive failure in the United States. Contraception 2011;83(5):398.

abortions, of whom 54% state that they were using contraception at the time they conceived. The vast majority of these method failures occurred with either condoms (28%) or pills (14%), whereas failures with LARC methods were uncommon at 1%.[13]

Satisfaction with a method is linked to continuation, which also influences contraceptive efficacy. One large cohort study found that at 1 year 86% of LARC users were continuing their method versus 55% of the short-acting method users.[6] At 2 years, 77% of LARC users were still using the method versus 41% of the short-acting method users.[5]

Women should retain the ability to change their contraceptive methods freely based on their preferences. Health care providers can help women who wish to discontinue a LARC method find another suitable method. They may not have this opportunity when women self-discontinue the pill, patch, or ring.

BARRIERS TO USING LONG-ACTING REVERSIBLE CONTRACEPTION

LARC use varies by method and country location. Globally, subdermal implants are underused despite their excellent efficacy; fewer than 1% of reproductive age women worldwide use implants for contraception. Even in countries with the highest uptake, rates are only 5% to 6%.[14] In contrast, 30% to 40% of reproductive age women in many Asian countries, like China, South Korea, and Viet Nam, rely on IUDs for contraception. Still other countries, including the United States, Canada, England, and Australia, report less than 10% of reproductive age women using an IUD.[14]

In the United States, relatively low rates of IUD use are partly related to misconceptions about safety of the IUD. In the 1970s, use of the Dalkon Shield was found to increase the risk of pelvic infections and subsequent infertility, resulting in a marked decrease in IUD use.[15] However, the legacy of the Dalkon Shield alone does not explain low rates of IUD use in the United States. Other barriers occur at the level of the patient, providers, and health care systems (**Table 2**).

Women

The decision for a woman to use any contraceptive method can be complex. Although patients accept that they should take medications to treat an illness, choosing to use

Table 2
Barriers to LARC use

Women	Providers
Undereducated about contraceptive options	Misperceptions about IUD use in adolescents
Misperceptions about safety of contraceptive methods	Misperceptions about IUD use in nulliparous women
Misperceptions about efficacy of contraceptive methods	Misperceptions about IUD use in women with a history of STI/PID
Feelings of invulnerability to getting pregnant	Misperceptions of IUD as abortifacient
Perception of subfertility	Misperceptions of implant risks
Ambivalence about pregnancy	Limited training on insertion techniques
Perception of low reproductive control	Fear of litigation
Male partner coercion	Fear of inadequate reimbursements

Abbreviations: IUD, intrauterine device; LARC, long-acting reversible contraception; STI, sexually transmitted infection.

contraception involves an interplay between the desire for pregnancy avoidance and the influences of intimacy, sexuality, and relationship negotiation. Some women have a direct attitude toward controlling their fertility, and others navigate a complicated web of factors. Two important elements in this decision-making process are intention and knowledge.

Pregnancy intention involves knowing one's reproductive desires as well as having the ability to control one's reproductive outcomes. In a recent qualitative study of low-income women in Pittsburgh, investigators found that many women did not perceive that they had reproductive control, and therefore did not conceptualize their pregnancy intentions.[16] One-third of the women in the study (32%) reported male partner coercion, ranging from verbal pressure to contraceptive sabotage. These women were not aware of the potential benefits of a planned pregnancy to both mother and baby, so planning pregnancy seemed less important. They were able to articulate which things they felt should be in place for the "ideal" timing of a pregnancy, regarding relationship and financial stability. However, few of the women surveyed were able to attain those ideals before pregnancy.[16] Clearly, in many instances women who are not interested in a pregnancy are not using any form of contraception. Such incongruous behavior may stem from a sense of lack of reproductive control.[16]

Pregnancy ambivalence can also be quite high. One study of 774 men and women aged 18 to 29 years old in relationships queried respondents about how strongly they wanted to avoid a pregnancy now, and how upset they would be if the woman became pregnant right now. Overall, 44.6% were ambivalent, with 53% of men and 36% of women reporting ambivalence, which correlated with lower use of any form of contraception.[17]

Women's knowledge about reproduction and their own fertility varies. Some qualitative studies have examined the attitudes of women seeking abortions toward unprotected intercourse. Common themes that emerged were a feeling of invulnerability to getting pregnant, because they had not gotten pregnant when having unprotected sex in the past, or a perceived level of subfertility.[18,19] Among 1392 women who had never had an abortion and were presenting for family planning services, 42% reported unprotected intercourse in the previous 3 months. Apart from problems accessing contraception, the other most common responses were not planning to have sex (45%) and perceived infertility (42%).[20]

Lack of knowledge about the full range of contraceptive options also influences contraceptive behavior. For many women, the word "contraception" is synonymous with the birth control pill. Other women may be aware of various contraceptive options, but do not understand their safety and efficacy. In a survey of 1665 women in the St. Louis area, a minority of women (28%) had discussed IUDs with their health care providers. Many women had misperceptions about the safety of the IUD, citing a risk of infection, infertility, and other problems. Additionally, women tended to underestimate the efficacy of the IUD or the implant, while overestimating the efficacy of pills, patches, ring, or condoms.[21]

The controversy over comprehensive sex education has led many school districts to provide just abstinence-only education, adversely affecting the contraceptive knowledge of teens in the United States. Although 91% of teens have some formal sex education on contraception and abstinence, only 70% of female teens have formal education that includes contraceptive methods. One-third (33%) of female teens reported coitarche before receiving formal sex education.[22,23] Studies show that only 31% to 45% of adolescents have ever heard of IUDs.[24] In 2009, only 4.5% of teens were using LARC.[2]

Providers

Inadequate knowledge regarding the benefits of LARC among health care providers creates a barrier to LARC use. Many providers have misconceptions about the safety of IUDs, and are reluctant to use IUDs in young and nulliparous women because of fear of pelvic inflammatory disease.[25–27] More than 80% of obstetricians/gynecologists in 1 survey advise against IUD use in women who are not monogamous, or who have a history of pelvic inflammatory disease.[28] A recent survey of 1150 fellows of the American College of Obstetrics and Gynecology (ACOG) revealed that only 43.0% thought IUDs were appropriate for adolescents, and just 30.0% thought IUDs were appropriate for women with a history of a sexually transmitted infection.[25] Additionally, more than 15% of those surveyed believed that pelvic inflammatory disease was a great risk for women with an IUD in place.[25]

Difficulty of insertion and pain during insertion are also mentioned frequently by health care providers as barriers to using IUDs in nulliparous women.[29] Lack of experience or infrequent insertion of IUDs in nulliparous women may influence a provider's confidence in insertion, and thus the decision to recommend the method.[30]

Misperceptions about the mechanism of action of IUDs may prevent some providers from using them. Among ACOG fellows who do not insert IUDs, about one-quarter of them stated the reason is they believe them to be an abortifacient.[31] An earlier study of ACOG members found that 20% agreed with the statement that IUDs are abortifacients.[28]

Fear of litigation may be a barrier to IUD use; 16% of ACOG members felt providing IUDs may increase their risk of a lawsuit.[28] US Food and Drug Administration packaging inserts on the LARC devices may also deter some physicians from using them. The copper IUD (Paragard, Teva) and newer levonorgestrel IUDs (Skyla, Bayer and Liletta, medicines360/Actavis) have received FDA approval for use in nulliparous women, but not the most widely used levonorgestrel IUD (Mirena, Bayer) does not. Most off-label use of drugs or devices does not have any legal or malpractice implications. However, most patients assume that any treatment they receive is FDA approved for that indication, and there is debate whether consent should be obtained for all off-label use, and whether it may impact people's perception of harm and their trust in providers.[32]

Misinformation also limits use of contraceptive implants. A survey of clinics in California providing family planning services to low-income women found that 16% thought smoking and 14% thought hypertension was a contraindication for implant use.[33]

Gaps in knowledge about IUDs and implants translate into suboptimal provision of contraceptive services to women. Although almost all ACOG fellows prescribe oral contraceptive pills (98.4%), only 91.8% insert the LNG IUD, 87.8% insert the copper IUD, and only 51.3% of those surveyed insert the contraceptive implant.[31] Of those providers who do place implants, only 60% had inserted an implant during the past year.[31] Almost one-third (31.7%) of ACOG fellows surveyed cited lack of insertion training as a reason for not providing implants.[31] In the California family planning clinic survey, just 65% of the clinics provided IUDs on site, and only 41% provided implants.[33]

Health Care Systems

Cost is clearly among the largest barriers to LARC use at the system level, affecting both patients and providers. Up-front costs of the device, combined with clinic visit and insertion fees, can be prohibitively expensive for a woman who is uninsured. The costs may total $1000 or more.[34] Even for women with insurance, the out-of-pocket costs can vary. One study showed that women with an out-of-pocket cost of $50 or less were more than 11 times more likely to have an IUD inserted than women with expenses of more than $500.[35] Another study found that women in the highest quartile of out of pocket costs for IUDs were 35% less likely to have an IUD inserted than in women in the lowest quartile of costs.[36] The Affordable Care Act will help to eliminate these discrepancies, because all FDA-approved contraceptive options should be available to women without cost sharing. However, not all insurance plans are in compliance with the Affordable Care Act, and several exemptions to coverage may make full implementation of the Affordable Care Act challenging.[37]

Cost to the provider is another systemic barrier to IUD provision. Providers may not insert LARC if they feel they will not be reimbursed adequately to even recoup the cost of the device. In the recent survey of obstetricians and gynecologists, one-third (33.3%) of those not providing IUDs and 27.9% of those not providing implants stated they would be more likely to do so if reimbursement were better.[31]

Timing and location of LARC insertion also influence provision practices. LARC may be placed at any time one can be reasonably certain that the woman is not pregnant, including immediately postpartum and after an abortion. Women should have access to LARC in outpatient offices, family planning clinics, operating rooms, labor and delivery, and postpartum wards.

For interval LARC insertion, same-day insertions can save the woman time and money. Requiring a 2-visit protocol may prevent a significant proportion (45.6%) of women from returning to the clinic to have the IUD inserted.[38] However, more than three-quarters of the ACOG fellows require 2 visits, and only 13% will insert an IUD in just 1 visit.[31] Reasons cited by clinicians for not providing same day LARC insertion include the need to have an up-to-date pap, prior testing for sexually transmitted infections, adequate time for counseling,[39] and insurance authorization.

Immediate postabortion IUD insertion has been shown to be safe and effective, with significantly more women relying on them at 6 months after an abortion than women who plan insertion at a follow-up visit.[40–42] Many clinics do not offer same-day insertions, citing several reasons. High cost for LARC insertion is a barrier for women, many of whom are already paying out of pocket for the abortion, and for providers who fear inadequate reimbursement.[43] Perceived lack of time for counseling and insertion without interrupting clinic flow, and lack of a protocol for immediate IUD insertion are additional barriers to postabortion LARC provision.[43] States that lack contraceptive coverage mandates have lower postabortion provision of LARC, as well as states with lesser Medicaid reimbursements for LARC.[43]

The availability of IUDs and implants in the immediate postpartum period can also increase access to effective contraception in women who are motivated to avoid pregnancy. If a method is not initiated before hospital discharge, many fail to return for a postpartum visit, consider alternate but less effective methods, or become pregnant before having a LARC inserted.[44] However, most insurance payments for delivery-related care are covered by a global fee, which in most states does not include initiation of LARC during the hospital stay.[45] In addition to cost, other institutional barriers include prohibitions to LARC insertion by Catholic hospitals, which account for a significant number of hospital beds; inadequate stocking of devices by in-patient pharmacies; and lack of trained personnel available at all times.[45]

RESULTS OF INCREASED USE OF LONG-ACTING REVERSIBLE CONTRACEPTION

There is a national movement to increase LARC use among women. Many organizations have endorsed LARC as a first line contraceptive option for all women including adolescents and nulliparous women (**Table 3**). Additionally, concentrated efforts to increase LARC use in particular regions have produced exciting results.

Regional initiatives
- Contraceptive CHOICE project, St Louis, Missouri
- Iowa Initiative to Reduce Unintended Pregnancies
- Colorado Family Planning Initiative

Contraceptive CHOICE Project

The Contraceptive CHOICE project enrolled more than 9000 women in the St. Louis area who received standardized, comprehensive contraceptive counseling and contraception free of cost for 3 years. Removing the barriers of cost and contraceptive knowledge resulted in three-quarters of the women in the cohort choosing a LARC method. Women using LARC were more satisfied with the method; had higher continuation rates than those using the pill, patch, or ring; and were less likely to have an unplanned pregnancy. Women using short-acting methods had 4.55 pregnancies per 100 woman-years of use, versus 0.27 pregnancies per 100 woman-years of LARC use.[4] Failure rates did not differ by age for LARC users, but adolescents (14–20 years of age) using short-acting methods were almost twice as likely to have an unintended pregnancy as older women using those methods.[4]

A large, St. Louis abortion clinic participating in the CHOICE project saw a 20.6% decrease in abortions. During the same time period no change occurred in the number of abortions in the rest of Missouri. The abortion rate among CHOICE participants was 4.4 to 7.5 per 1000 versus the regional rate of 13.4 to 17.0 per 1000, and the national rate of 19.6 per 1000.[9]

There was also a dramatic decrease in teen pregnancies. Similar to adult participants, 72% of teens in CHOICE chose a LARC method—37% IUDs and 35% implants. The

Table 3
Organizational position statements on use of LARC

Organization	Recommendations
American College of Obstetrician and Gynecologists (ACOG)	Offer LARC as first-line contraceptive option to most women, including adolescents and nulliparous women.[46,47]
	Launched LARC program—initiative to disseminate information, provide clinical training, e-learning, and webinars.
American Academy of Pediatrics (AAP)	LARC methods should be considered first-line contraceptive methods for adolescents.[48]
American Academy of Family Physicians (AAFP)	Encourage appropriate patients to use LARCs. Few contraindications, even in nulliparous women and adolescents.[49]
Center for Disease Control US Selective Practice Recommendations for Contraceptive Use (CDC–US SPR)	Contraceptive effectiveness important when choosing method. LARC is highly effective. LARC appropriate for most women, including adolescents and nulliparous women.[50]

Abbreviation: LARC, long-acting reversible contraception.
Data from Refs.[46–50]

pregnancy rate, birth rate, and abortion rate among teen participants all dropped to less than one-quarter the rates reported among sexually active US teens.[12]

Iowa

Iowa increased access to LARC for low-income women by state expansion of Medicaid-funded family planning services, as well as a privately funded initiative to increase funding for family planning services at several sites for low-income women. Over the course of 8 years, the use of LARC increased from less than 1% to 15% of women receiving care in these family planning clinics, compared with an increase from less than 0.10% to 1.5% in the general Iowan population. The 15% LARC users were equally divided between IUD and implant users. During the same time period, the number of abortions in the state declined, from 8.7 per 1000 reproductive age women to 6.7 per 1000. This decrease came within the context of expanded access to abortion services in Iowa.[11]

Colorado

The Colorado Family Planning Initiative was launched in 2009 in an effort to decrease unintended pregnancies, particularly in young women. Private funding was used to increase access to LARC via Title X family planning clinics in 2 ways: providing funds to purchase devices and training and support for staff. Over the next few years, a sharp increase in patients was seen; more than one-half under 25 years old, and the vast majority under the federal poverty level. LARC use increased from 4.5% to 19.4%, with 9% implants and 10.4% IUDs. This correlated with a statewide decrease in both birth rates and abortion rates. The birth rate decreased by 29% in teens 15 to 19 years old, and by 14% in 20 to 24 year olds. Similarly, the abortion rate decreased by 34% and 18% in these age groups, respectively.[10]

These 3 examples represent distinct populations across the country. The participants in CHOICE were predominantly African American and white in an urban environment[9]; presumably those in Iowa were predominantly white and rural, and in Colorado, more than 40% of the women attending the Title X clinics were Hispanic.[10] Such encouraging results suggest that it is not the region or the women, but the access to and education about LARC that impacts usage.

SUMMARY

The evidence is clear that LARC has superior efficacy to short-acting contraceptive methods. Women who use LARC tend to be more satisfied with their method and more likely to continue to use their method. LARC users are less likely to have an unplanned pregnancy than women using short-acting methods. Unfortunately, fewer than 10% of all reproductive age women using contraception in the United States are using LARC. Many barriers contribute to this poor LARC use, although none is unsurmountable. Recent interventions aimed at increasing the use of LARC have been successful, which has translated into lower rates of unplanned pregnancy. When women are given ample education and easy access to LARC, many more choose it and are satisfied.

Continued interventions must expand on several levels. We must better inform our patients about their contraceptive options. Simultaneously, we must educate or reeducate health care providers so they feel comfortable with the appropriate usage and insertion of LARC. Last, we must strive to prevent cost from influencing women's and providers' choice of contraceptive method. With increased use of LARC among reproductive age women, we may finally see a decrease in the rate of unplanned pregnancies in the United States.

REFERENCES

1. Finer LB, Zolna MR. Unintended pregnancy in the United States: incidence and disparities, 2006. Contraception 2011;84(5):478–85.
2. Finer LB, Jerman J, Kavanaugh ML. Changes in use of long-acting contraceptive methods in the United States, 2007–2009. Fertil Steril 2012;98(4):893–7.
3. Trussell J. Contraceptive failure in the United States. Contraception 2011;83(5): 397–404.
4. Winner B, Peipert JF, Zhao Q, et al. Effectiveness of long-acting reversible contraception. N Engl J Med 2012;366(21):1998–2007.
5. O'Neil-Callahan M, Peipert JF, Zhao Q, et al. Twenty-four-month continuation of reversible contraception. Obstet Gynecol 2013;122(5):1083–91.
6. Peipert JF, Zhao Q, Allsworth JE, et al. Continuation and satisfaction of reversible contraception. Obstet Gynecol 2011;117(5):1105–13.
7. Rosenstock JR, Peipert JF, Madden T, et al. Continuation of reversible contraception in teenagers and young women. Obstet Gynecol 2012;120(6):1298–305.
8. Dickerson LM, Diaz VA, Jordon J, et al. Satisfaction, early removal, and side effects associated with long-acting reversible contraception. Fam Med 2013;45(10):701–7.
9. Peipert JF, Madden T, Allsworth JE, et al. Preventing unintended pregnancies by providing no-cost contraception. Obstet Gynecol 2012;120(6):1291–7.
10. Ricketts S, Klingler G, Schwalberg R. Game change in Colorado: widespread use of long-acting reversible contraceptives and rapid decline in births among young, low-income women. Perspect Sex Reprod Health 2014;46(3):125–32.
11. Biggs MA, Rocca CH, Brindis CD, et al. Did increasing use of highly effective contraception contribute to declining abortions in Iowa? Contraception 2015; 91(2):167–73.
12. Secura GM, Madden T, McNicholas C, et al. Provision of no-cost, long-acting contraception and teenage pregnancy. N Engl J Med 2014;371(14):1316–23.
13. Jones RK, Darroch JE, Henshaw SK. Contraceptive use among U.S. women having abortions in 2000-2001. Perspect Sex Reprod Health 2006;34(6):10.
14. United Nations PD. World contraceptive patterns 2013. 2013 [2/5/14]. Available at: www.un.org/en/development/desa/population/publications/pdf/family/world ContraceptivePatternsWallChart2013.pdf. Accessed February 5, 2014.
15. Sivin I. Another look at the Dalkon Shield: meta-analysis underscores its problems. Contraception 1993;48(1):1–12.
16. Borrero S, Nikolajski C, Steinberg JR, et al. "It just happens": a qualitative study exploring low-income women's perspectives on pregnancy intention and planning. Contraception 2015;91(2):150–6.
17. Higgins JA, Popkin RA, Santelli JS. Pregnancy ambivalence and contraceptive use among young adults in the United States. Perspect Sex Reprod Health 2012;44(4):236–43.
18. Foster DG, Higgins JA, Karasek D, et al. Attitudes toward unprotected intercourse and risk of pregnancy among women seeking abortion. Womens Health Issues 2012;22(2):e149–55.
19. Frohwirth L, Moore AM, Maniaci R. Perceptions of susceptibility to pregnancy among U.S. women obtaining abortions. Soc Sci Med 2013;99:18–26.
20. Biggs MA, Karasek D, Foster DG. Unprotected intercourse among women wanting to avoid pregnancy: attitudes, behaviors, and beliefs. Womens Health Issues 2012;22(3):e311–8.
21. Hladky KJ, Allsworth JE, Madden T, et al. Women's knowledge about intrauterine contraception. Obstet Gynecol 2011;117(1):48–54.

22. McCracken KA, Loveless M. Teen pregnancy: an update. Curr Opin Obstet Gynecol 2014;26(5):355–9.
23. Facts on American Teens' Sources of Information about Sex 2012 [June 19, 2015]. Available at: www.guttmacher.org/pubs/FB-Teen-Sex-Ed.html#12. Accessed June 19, 2015.
24. Teal SB, Romer SE. Awareness of Long-Acting Reversible Contraception Among Teens and Young Adults. J Adolesc Health 2013;52(4, Suppl):S35–9.
25. Luchowski AT, Anderson BL, Power ML, et al. Obstetrician-gynecologists and contraception: practice and opinions about the use of IUDs in nulliparous women, adolescents and other patient populations. Contraception 2014; 89(6):572–7.
26. Tyler CP, Whiteman MK, Zapata LB, et al. Health care provider attitudes and practices related to intrauterine devices for nulliparous women. Obstet Gynecol 2012; 119(4):762–71.
27. Harper CC, Blum M, de Bocanegra HT, et al. Challenges in translating evidence to practice: the provision of intrauterine contraception. Obstet Gynecol 2008; 111(6):1359–69.
28. Stanwood NL, Garrett JM, Konrad TR. Obstetrician-gynecologists and the intrauterine device: a survey of attitudes and practice. Obstet Gynecol 2002;99(2): 275–80.
29. Black KI, Lotke P, Lira J, et al. Global survey of healthcare practitioners' beliefs and practices around intrauterine contraceptive method use in nulliparous women. Contraception 2013;88(5):650–6.
30. Gilmore K, Hoopes AJ, Cady J, et al. Providing long-acting reversible contraception services in Seattle school-based health centers: key themes for facilitating implementation. J Adolesc Health 2015;56(6):658–65.
31. Luchowski AT, Anderson BL, Power ML, et al. Obstetrician-gynecologists and contraception: long-acting reversible contraception practices and education. Contraception 2014;89(6):578–83.
32. Legro RS. Introduction: on-label and off-label drug use in reproductive medicine. Fertil Steril 2015;103(3):581–2.
33. Biggs MAP, Harper CCP, Malvin JP, et al. Factors influencing the provision of long-acting reversible contraception in California. Obstet Gynecol 2014;123(3): 593–602.
34. Eisenberg D, McNicholas C, Peipert JF. Cost as a barrier to long-acting reversible contraceptive (LARC) use in adolescents. J Adolesc Health 2013;52(4 Suppl): S59–63.
35. Gariepy AM, Simon EJ, Patel DA, et al. The impact of out-of-pocket expense on IUD utilization among women with private insurance. Contraception 2011;84(6): e39–42.
36. Pace LE, Dusetzina SB, Fendrick AM, et al. The impact of out-of-pocket costs on the use of intrauterine contraception among women with employer-sponsored insurance. Med Care 2013;51(11):959–63.
37. Insurance coverage of contraceptives. Guttmacher Institute, 2015.
38. Bergin A, Tristan S, Terplan M, et al. A missed opportunity for care: two-visit IUD insertion protocols inhibit placement. Contraception 2012;86(6):694–7.
39. Biggs MA, Arons A, Turner R, et al. Same-day LARC insertion attitudes and practices. Contraception 2013;88(5):629–35.
40. Fox MC, Oat-Judge J, Severson K, et al. Immediate placement of intrauterine devices after first and second trimester pregnancy termination. Contraception 2011; 83(1):34–40.

41. Cremer M, Bullard KA, Mosley RM, et al. Immediate vs. delayed post-abortal copper T 380A IUD insertion in cases over 12 weeks of gestation. Contraception 2011;83(6):522–7.
42. Bednarek PH, Creinin MD, Reeves MF, et al. Immediate versus delayed IUD insertion after uterine aspiration. N Engl J Med 2011;364(23):2208–17.
43. Thompson KMJ, Speidel JJ, Saporta V, et al. Contraceptive policies affect post-abortion provision of long-acting reversible contraception. Contraception 2011; 83(1):41–7.
44. Ogburn JA, Espey E, Stonehocker J. Barriers to intrauterine device insertion in postpartum women. Contraception 2005;72(6):426–9.
45. Aiken ARA, Creinin MD, Kaunitz AM, et al. Global fee prohibits postpartum provision of the most effective reversible contraceptives. Contraception 2014; 90(5):466–7.
46. American College of Obstetricians and Gynecologists Committee on Gynecologic Practice, Long-Acting Reversible Contraception Working Group. ACOG Committee Opinion No. 450: increasing use of contraceptive implants and intrauterine devices to reduce unintended pregnancy. Obstet Gynecol 2009;114(6): 1434–8.
47. Committee on Adolescent Health Care Long-Acting Reversible Contraception Working Group, The American College of Obstetricians and Gynecologists. Committee Opinion No. 539: adolescents and long-acting reversible contraception: implants and intrauterine devices. Obstet Gynecol 2012;120(4):983–8.
48. Committee on Adolescence. Contraception for adolescents. Pediatrics 2014; 134(4):e1244–56.
49. Randel A. Guidelines for the use of long-acting reversible contraceptives. Am Fam Physician 2012;85(4):403–4.
50. Division of Reproductive Health, National Center for Chronic Disease Prevention and Health Promotion, Centers for Disease Control and Prevention (CDC). U.S. Selected Practice Recommendations for Contraceptive Use, 2013: adapted from the World Health Organization selected practice recommendations for contraceptive use, 2nd edition. MMWR Recomm Rep 2013;62(RR-05):1–60.

Immediate Postpartum Intrauterine Contraception Insertion

Sarah W. Prager, MD, MAS*, Erin E. McCoy, MPH

KEYWORDS

- Postpartum period • Intrauterine devices • Contraceptive agents • Female • Copper
- Levonorgestrel

KEY POINTS

- The immediate postpartum period is a favorable time for initiating contraception, given high levels of motivation to use contraception after delivery, convenience for patients and physicians, and the fact that pregnancy is excluded.
- Immediate postpartum intrauterine contraception (PPIUC) is safe and effective and a majority of intrauterine contraception (IUC) devices are retained.
- Increased rates of device expulsion compared with delayed postpartum insertion and interval insertion have been demonstrated. This risk should be weighed against the risk of patients not returning at all for postpartum follow-up.
- Although immediate PPIUC may not be the right choice for all women in every clinical setting, it remains a reasonable choice for many.

INTRODUCTION TO IMMEDIATE POSTPARTUM INTRAUTERINE CONTRACEPTION

The immediate postpartum period is a favorable time for initiating contraception, because women who have recently given birth are often highly motivated to use contraception, pregnancy is excluded, and the hospital setting offers convenience for both patients and the health care providers. This article addresses both the copper IUC and the 52-mg levonorgestrel (LNG) intrauterine system (IUS) (Mirena [Bayer, NJ, USA]). There are no published data on immediate postpartum use of the lower dose 13.5-mg LNG-IUS (Skyla [Bayer, NJ, USA]) or the new 52-mg LNG-IUS (Liletta [Actavis, NJ, USA]), so all references to LNG-IUS in this article are to the 52-mg LNG-IUS (Mirena).

Disclosure Statement: S.W. Prager trains providers in Nexplanon insertion and removal (receives no honoraria). E.E. McCoy has nothing to disclose.
Department of Obstetrics and Gynecology, University of Washington, Box 356460, Seattle, WA 98195, USA
* Corresponding author.
E-mail address: pragers@uw.edu

Obstet Gynecol Clin N Am 42 (2015) 569–582
http://dx.doi.org/10.1016/j.ogc.2015.08.001
0889-8545/15/$ – see front matter © 2015 Elsevier Inc. All rights reserved.

WHAT IS POSTPARTUM INTRAUTERINE CONTRACEPTION?

Many providers of contraception are unaware that placement of IUC immediately after delivery is possible. The following terms describe the timing of placement of the IUC:

- Postplacental IUC refers to the placement of IUC within 10 minutes of delivery of the placenta.
- Immediate PPIUC refers to the placement of IUC within the first 48 hours after delivery.
- Immediate postcesarean IUC refers to the placement of IUC through the hysterotomy at the time of cesarean delivery.
- Delayed postpartum IUC is placed typically 4 to 6 weeks postpartum.
- Interval placement—IUC placement not related to timing of childbirth.

The timing of placement can have relevance to rates of expulsion as well as implementation consequences for programs. This is discussed later.

WHY PLACE POSTPARTUM INTRAUTERINE CONTRACEPTION?

Immediate PPIUC placement has several major advantages over interval insertion. First, confirmation that a woman is not pregnant is a necessary requirement prior to IUC insertion. The immediate postpartum period offers complete certainty of this requirement.

Second, women are usually in the care of a health care provider at the time of delivery. In the United States, as in all industrialized countries, nearly all deliveries occur within a hospital. Of the 1.36% of births that took place outside a hospital in the United States in 2012,[1] 99% of these are attended by a skilled birth attendant (SBA). Although a lower proportion of deliveries take place with the presence of an SBA in low- and middle-resource settings, globally, the proportion of births attended by skilled birth personnel increased from 59% to 68% between 1990 and 2009.[2]

Delivery by an SBA is increasing globally, but access to contraceptive care is often limited. Some women face significant geographic barriers to accessing care, let alone access to a provider trained in placing IUC. Other women lack the financial resources to get to a clinic or provider. Still others simply do not have the time, given work and/or family responsibilities. For all these women, placement of IUC before they leave the hospital after delivery allows them to manage their contraception without any additional visits. Many women who would not follow-up after IUC placement alone may follow-up with a provider after delivery for either themselves or their newborn child.[3,4] This increases the chance of evaluating PPIUC within 2 to 6 weeks and addressing any concerns or complications.

The availability of equipment and skilled personnel at the time of delivery allows for additional convenience with immediate PPIUC insertion. To place immediate PPIUC, all that is needed are the following (**Fig. 1**):

- 1 To 2 ring forceps
- Cotton swabs or gauze
- Sterile gloves
- Povidone Iodine or another antiseptic
- Right-angle retractor (not always needed)
- Scissors/razor (not always needed – depends on type of IUC)
- IUC

All necessary items are normally present or immediately available at the time of a vaginal or cesarean delivery, so no additional equipment is required.

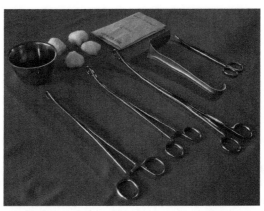

Fig. 1. Equipment needed for immediate PPIUC insertion. (*Courtesy of* Cardea Services, Seattle, Washington; with permission.)

Also present on a labor ward or postpartum unit are health care providers skilled in pelvic examination. If these health care providers are not already experienced in IUC insertion, they can be trained to perform this procedure. Many low-resource settings have few health care providers per capita and even fewer physicians. Approximately 44% of World Health Organization member states report to have less than 1 physician per 1000 population.[5] These numbers do not reflect the numbers of nonphysician medical professionals who also contribute to patient care; in almost all countries, nursing and midwifery services are estimated to comprise more than 80% of the health care services.[5] There always are labor nurses, midwives, and either obstetricians or other general physicians present at a hospital or facility that does deliveries. It is also somewhat easier to target IUC trainings to sites that do deliveries, because these providers are also generally more likely to be motivated to perform women's health care.

A final barrier that is automatically overcome by immediate PPIUC is the closed cervix. For providers, a closed cervix can make an interval IUC insertion more challenging, more likely to result in a complication, or simply impossible to perform. With interval insertion, pain is a concern for many women. Qualitative studies have identified fear about the insertion procedure as a barrier to IUD use.[6,7] Predictors of pain during IUD insertion include nulliparity, age greater than 30 years, longer time since last pregnancy or last menses, nonlactation,[8] and psychosocial factors.[9,10] Self-reported pain scores with interval IUC insertion vary significantly.[11] Mean levels of pain at time of insertion were significantly greater for procedures more than 3 months since time of last delivery.[8] Studies on pain management techniques during the procedure have been limited and results have been conflicting.

No study has directly compared pain with PPIUC versus interval insertion. Pain with PPIUC has been compared with delayed postpartum insertion. In 1 study, 80% of the subjects who were randomized to receive immediate PPIUC with LNG-IUS reported no or mild pain with insertion. In the late postpartum insertion group, 88% reported no to mild pain, although there was some loss to follow-up in that group.[12] Removing the barrier of a separate, potentially uncomfortable procedure can be attractive to both patients and providers.

HOW IS AN IMMEDIATE POSTPARTUM INTRAUTERINE CONTRACEPTION PLACED?

Placement of PPIUC at the time of vaginal delivery can be done using the IUC inserter, a ring forceps or other holding instrument, or simply a provider's hand (**Fig. 2**). When

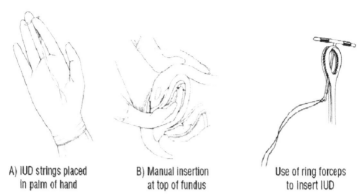

A) IUD strings placed   B) Manual insertion   Use of ring forceps
   in palm of hand   at top of fundus   to Insert IUD

Fig. 2. Two techniques of postplacental IUD insertion and proper location of IUD after insertion. (*Courtesy of* EngenderHealth, New York, NY; with permission.)

hand insertion of a copper IUC was compared with insertion with a ring forceps, no differences in efficacy or infection emerged (although this, and other, studies are underpowered to detect a real difference in the low rate of infection).[13]

Studies have not addressed differences in discomfort with different methods of placement nor have they investigated differences in levels of pain experienced by women who receive pain medications intrapartum versus those who were unmedicated.

Efficacy using the prepackaged IUD inserters has also not been assessed. There are no studies looking at the copper IUC inserter, because it is typically too short to reach the fundus of a postpartum uterus. Studies of the LNG-IUS vary on methodology, using the LNG-IUS inserter, ring forceps, or hand insertion but have not directly compared the methods.[3,12]

Preinsertion Tasks
- Assess for eligibility (discussed later).
- Perform bimanual examination.
- Clean the external genital area with a clean cloth.
- Place a clean drape over the client's abdomen and underneath her buttocks.
- Change gloves.

Pelvic Examination
- Insert a speculum, retractor, or gloved hand into the vagina and visualize the cervix.
- Clean the cervix and the vagina with antiseptic solution (not evidence based).
- Gently grasp the anterior lip of the cervix with ring forceps. (Do not use a toothed tenaculum because it may tear the cervix.)

Instrument Insertion: Copper Intrauterine Contraception
- Grasp the IUC with Kelly Placenta Forceps (**Fig. 3**) or with a second pair of standard ring forceps (**Fig. 4**).
- The IUC should be held by its vertical stem; the horizontal arm of the IUC should be just above the ring and in the same plane.
- The ring should be slightly eccentrically placed so the distal tip of the stem is NOT within the ring.
- The eccentric placement facilitates the liberation of the IUC in the fundus, decreasing the risk of pulling it out while removing the forceps.

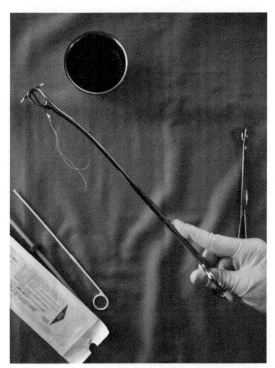

Fig. 3. IUC handled with Kelly Placenta Forceps. (*Courtesy of* Cardea Services, Seattle, WA; with permission.)

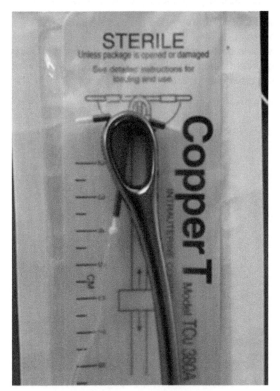

Fig. 4. Loading the IUC within the package. (*Courtesy of* Cardea Services, Seattle, WA; with permission.)

- Exert gentle traction on the cervix-holding forceps (**Fig. 5**).
- Insert the forceps holding the IUC through the cervix and into the lower uterine cavity. Avoid touching the walls of the vagina with the IUC.
- As the IUC passes through the cervix, release the hand that is holding the cervix-holding forceps and move this hand to the abdomen, placing it over the uterine fundus.
- With the abdominal hand, stabilize the uterus with firm downward pressure through the abdominal wall. Prevent the uterus from moving upward in the abdomen as the IUC is inserted (**Fig. 6**).
- Move the IUC-holding forceps toward the fundus (in an angle toward the umbilicus) (**Fig. 7**).
- Remember that the lower uterine segment may be contracted and, therefore, some slight pressure may be necessary to advance the IUD and achieve fundal placement.
- By feeling the uterus through the relaxed abdominal wall, confirm with the abdominal hand that the tips of the forceps reach the fundus.
- If the client has delivered vaginally after a previous cesarean delivery, take care to avoid placing the IUC through any defect in the previous incision by maintaining the ring forceps pressure against the posterior uterine wall.
- At the fundus, turn the forceps so that the IUC is in the proper horizontal orientation (**Fig. 8**).
- Open the forceps, releasing the IUC.
- Slowly remove the forceps from the uterine cavity, keeping it slightly open, and sweeping the forceps slightly laterally to avoid entanglement with the strings.

Postinsertion Tasks: Copper Intrauterine Contraception
- Examine the cervix.
- IUC strings should be at or above the external os and should not need cutting.
- If there is significant string length seen, the IUC may not be at fundus.
- Remove the cervix-holding forceps from the anterior lip of the cervix.

Insertion: Levonorgestrel–Intrauterine Contraception
Option 1
- Keep LNG-IUC in the inserter.

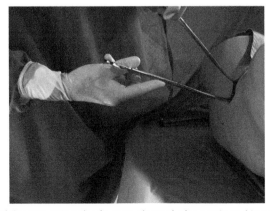

Fig. 5. Insertion of the IUC, using the forceps, through the cervix and into the lower uterine cavity. (*Courtesy of* Cardea Services, Seattle, WA; with permission.)

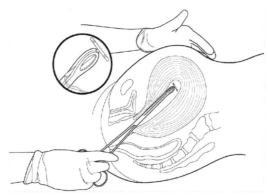

Fig. 6. Place a hand on the uterine fundus to assist in high fundal placement of the IUC. (*Courtesy of* Tracy Angulo, BA, Seattle, WA, 2011.)

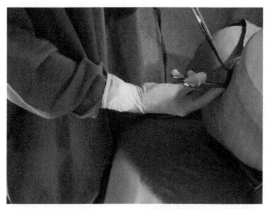

Fig. 7. Move the IUC-holding forceps toward the fundus in an angle toward the umbilicus. (*Courtesy of* Cardea Services, Seattle, WA; with permission.)

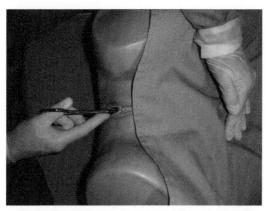

Fig. 8. At the fundus, turn the forceps so that the IUC is in the proper horizontal orientation, and open the forceps to release the IUC. (*Courtesy of* Cardea Services, Seattle, WA; with permission.)

- Do not load the arms of the "T" – they can stay outside of the inserter.
- Follow all other steps as with copper IUC.
- Release at the fundus and gently check that the IUC feels like it is at the fundus.
- Cut the strings at the external os.

Option 2

- Remove IUC from inserter.
- *Gently* hold IUC in forceps *without locking*.
- Place according to copper IUC instructions.
- Precut the strings to 10–25 cm.

Manual Insertion Technique

- Visualize the cervix with the aid of a retractor.
- A long sleeve sterile pair of gloves or standard gloves WITH water-impermeable gown are needed.
- Use a hand, rather than forceps, to insert the IUC (**Fig. 9**).
- Hold the IUC by gripping the vertical stem between the index and middle fingers of the predominant hand (**Fig. 10**).
- Insert the IUC-holding hand into the vagina and through the cervix into the uterus (**Fig. 11**).
- Direct the IUC toward the abdominal hand, which should be firmly holding the uterine fundus through the relaxed abdominal wall (**Fig. 12**).
- Stabilize the uterus by downward pressure to prevent it going up higher in the abdomen as the IUC-holding hand is inserted.
- Confirm by palpation with the external hand that the fundus has been reached.
- Take particular care not to dislodge the IUC as the hand is slowly removed from the uterus.

Key Points with Postpartum Intrauterine Contraception Insertion

- Place hand on fundus
  - Confirms high fundal placement
  - Reduces/eliminates chance of perforation
  - Helps provider know where to aim

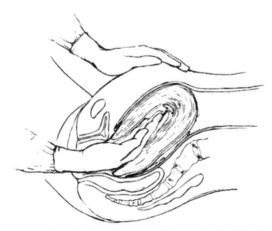

Fig. 9. Insert the IUC with a hand. (*Courtesy of* EngenderHealth, New York, NY; with permission.)

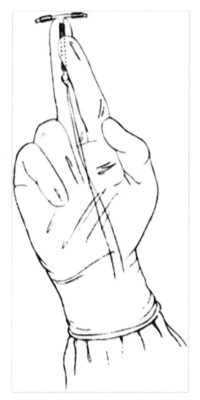

Fig. 10. Hold the IUC by gripping the vertical stem between the index and middle fingers of the predominant hand. (*Courtesy of* EngenderHealth, New York, NY; with permission.)

- Direct the forceps straight up toward abdominal wall/umbilicus.
  - Not toward the head
  - Drop the wrist
- Know the orientation of the IUD with respect to the orientation of the forceps.

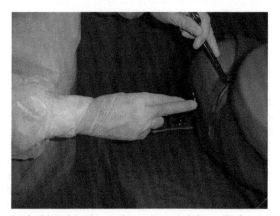

Fig. 11. Insert the IUC-holding hand into the vagina and through the cervix into the uterus. (*Courtesy of* Cardea Services, Seattle, WA; with permission.)

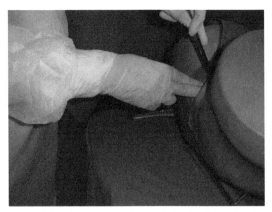

Fig. 12. Direct the IUC-holding hand toward the abdominal hand, which should be firmly holding the uterine fundus through the relaxed abdominal wall. (*Courtesy of* Cardea Services, Seattle, WA; with permission.)

- Cut strings at external os (if indicated).
  - Different length strings with different IUC devices
  - Different depths of postpartum uterus

WHAT IS THE RATE OF EXPULSION WITH IMMEDIATE POSTPARTUM INTRAUTERINE CONTRACEPTION?

The main concern with immediate PPIUC is expulsion. Expulsion rates for interval IUC placement range from 0% to 11%, with no real differences seen between IUC devices.[14–16] Parous women, and those aged 14 to 19, do have increased rates of expulsion compared with nulliparous women and those aged 20 and older, comparatively.[16] All studies of immediate PPIUC report higher expulsion rates than those found with interval or delayed postpartum insertion. A systematic review of PPIUC with a copper device found the expulsion rate for postcesarean insertion was less than with postplacental insertion after vaginal delivery, which is then less than delayed postpartum placement.[17] A recent study of the copper T380 A in Uganda, which randomized women to immediate postcesarean versus delayed postpartum, found 100% placement rates in the immediate arm versus 53% placement rate in the delayed arm ($P<.0001$).[18] Using intention-to-treat analysis, this same study found 6-month retention of IUC to be 79% in the immediate arm versus 47% in the delayed arm ($P<.01$), with no difference in expulsion rates.[18] Another study of postplacental copper T380A device insertion in women who delivered vaginally (74% subjects) or at time of cesarean delivery (26% subjects) found expulsion rates of 5.1% at 6 weeks, 7% at 6 months, and 12.3% at 12 months.[19] An early study of immediate PPIUC with various nonhormonal IUC devices, none of which is commonly used now, pooled data from several centers around the world. The adjusted pooled analysis shows an expulsion rate of 9.3% with placement less than 10 minutes after placental expulsion, 31.5% with placement at 2 to 23 hours postpartum, 37.3% at 24 to 47 hours postpartum, and 28.8% at 48 to 72 hours postpartum.[20] This same analysis showed differential rates of expulsion at 6 months depending on whether subjects were recruited during the first or second half of the study period: 12% versus 6.9%, respectively.[20] This indicates that provider experience may play a significant role in reducing the rate of expulsion.

Studies using the LNG-IUS are more recent than many of the studies of PPIUC using copper IUC, although they have fewer subjects. One study randomized women to immediate postplacental versus 6-week delayed insertion of LNG-IUS. Ultrasound guidance was used, as was the LNG-IUS inserter. Expulsion rates were 24.4% versus 4.4% (P = .008) for postplacental and delayed insertions, respectively.[12] A study randomizing subjects to immediate postcesarean versus 4- to 8-week delayed insertion of LNG-IUS found 20% versus 0% expulsion rates (P = .04).[3] Even with different expulsion rates, confirmed use at 12 months was similar in both groups, with a similar loss to follow-up.[3] To date, no studies, including both LNG-IUS and copper IUC devices, have had enough power to directly compare immediate postpartum expulsion rates; however, expulsion may be more common with LNG-IUS than with copper IUC. It is unclear if this is due to the different IUC shapes or materials or some other factor. Data are lacking comparing insertion of LNG-IUS using the prepackaged inserter versus using a ring or other forceps instrument versus hand insertion.

WHAT ARE OTHER COMPLICATIONS WITH IMMEDIATE POSTPARTUM INTRAUTERINE CONTRACEPTION?

In addition to expulsion, the other complications of concern are perforation, infection, and bleeding complications. No study using any IUC device has found increased risks of perforation with PPIUC versus delayed or interval placement.[3,12,17,21] Newer data show a 6-fold increased risk of perforation with delayed postpartum IUC placement versus interval insertion with both LNG-IUS and copper IUC (absolute risk differences were 5 more perforations per 1000 women using the LNG-IUS and 2 more perforations per 1000 women using the copper IUC).[22] This cohort did not include women having immediate PPIUC insertion. These data should not discourage providers from placing IUC at a 6-week postpartum visit, only to use more caution and to support the safety of immediate PPIUC where essentially no perforations have been reported.

Higher infection rates have not been reported in studies of PPIUC at any time after delivery or after any mode of delivery.[3,12,17,21] Rates of infection are low overall, so many studies are not powered to find this difference.

Bleeding irregularities have also not been found problematic in women choosing immediate PPIUC.[3,17,21] The amenorrhea associated with breastfeeding postpartum may mask bleeding irregularities.

HOW TO DECIDE IF A PATIENT IS APPROPRIATE FOR IMMEDIATE POSTPARTUM INTRAUTERINE CONTRACEPTION

All women should receive contraception counseling during pregnancy. Counseling should include a discussion of immediate PPIUC placement for anyone indicating a desire for IUC after delivery. The Centers for Disease Control Medical Eligibility Criteria for Contraceptive Use (CDC MEC) consider PPIUC at any time point, with any IUC, category 1 to 2 (1 = no restrictions and 2 = benefits generally outweigh the theoretic or proved risks).[23] If a woman chooses to have immediate PPIUC, she still needs to meet certain criteria at the time of delivery. Recommendations include ascertaining risk of infection, so women with signs or symptoms of chorioamnionitis, or with prolonged rupture of membranes are generally not good candidates for PPIUC. The CDC MEC consider use of PPIUC category 4 (unacceptable health risk) in the presence of puerperal sepsis.[23] There are no data parsing out the various risks with length of ruptured membranes; however, the criteria listed in **Fig. 13** are generally used to determine eligibility for immediate PPIUC.

In preparation for insertion of the IUC, confirm the following information about the woman and her clinical situation:		
Ask the woman whether she still desires the IUC for immediate PPFP	☐ No	☐ Yes
Review her antenatal record and be certain that		
• Her antenatal screening shows that an IUC is an appropriate method for her	☐ No	☐ Yes
• She has had FP counseling while not in active labor and there is evidence of consent in her chart OR	☐ No	☐ Yes
• She is being counseled in the postpartum period	☐ No	☐ Yes

Review the course of her labor and delivery and ensure that none of the following conditions is present:		
If planning an *immediate postplacental insertion*, check whether any of the following conditions is present:		
• Chorioamnionitis (during labor)	☐ No	☐ Yes
• More than 18–24 hours from rupture of membranes to delivery of baby	☐ No	☐ Yes
• Unresolved postpartum hemorrhage	☐ No	☐ Yes

If planning an *immediate postpartum insertion*, check whether any of the following conditions is present:		
• Puerperal sepsis	☐ No	☐ Yes
• Postpartum endometritis/metritis	☐ No	☐ Yes
• Continued excessive postpartum bleeding	☐ No	☐ Yes
• Extensive genital trauma where the repair would be disrupted by immediate postpartum placement of an IUC	☐ No	☐ Yes

| *Confirm* that IUCs are available and accessible on the labor ward | ☐ No | ☐ Yes |

Fig. 13. Criteria generally used to determine eligibility for immediate PPIUC. If *ANY* BLUE box is checked "No" or RED box is checked "Yes", defer insertion of the IUC and provide the woman with information about another method. If *ALL* the BLUE boxes are checked "Yes" and the RED boxes are checked "No", then proceed with IUC insertion. FP, family planning; PPFP, postpartum family planning. (*Adapted from* Blumenthal P. Population Services International Training Guide. Palo Alto, CA. 2012.)

In summary, immediate PPIUC is safe and effective, with a majority of IUC devices retained at 6 and 12 months.[17,21] The rates of expulsion are increased compared with delayed postpartum insertion and interval insertion; however, this needs to be weighed against the risk of patients not returning for postpartum follow-up. In a population like that seen in Lester and colleagues' study in Uganda,[18] where only 53% of subjects randomized to the 6-week delayed postpartum insertion arm returned for their visit, accepting a higher rate of expulsion might be reasonable. In a population such as that seen in Whitaker and colleagues' study of postcesarean IUC,[3] where 70% to 100% of subjects returned for their delayed postpartum IUC insertion, providers can discuss with patients the merits and detractors of accepting a higher expulsion rate. Even in populations where postpartum follow-up is relatively high, immediate postpartum insertion can benefit an individual woman who faces barriers to follow-up or prefers postpartum insertion. A cost-effectiveness analysis of immediate PPIUC found that strategy would prevent 88 pregnancies per 1000 women over a 2-year period and is cost effective in 99% of all simulations.[24] Immediate PPIUC may not be the right choice for all women in every clinical setting; however, it remains a reasonable choice for many and should be included in the basic armamentarium of options for women.

REFERENCES

1. MacDorman MF, Matthews TJ, Declercq E. Trends in out-of-hospital births in the United States, 1990–2012. NCHS Data Brief 2014;(144):1–8.
2. Organization WHO. Trends in maternal mortality: 1990 to 2013. Estimates by WHO, UNICEF, UNFPA, The World Bank and the United Nations Population Division. Geneva (Switzerland): WHO; 2014.
3. Whitaker AK, Endres LK, Mistretta SQ, et al. Postplacental insertion of the levonorgestrel intrauterine device after cesarean delivery vs. delayed insertion: a randomized controlled trial. Contraception 2014;89(6):534–9.
4. Ogburn JA, Espey E, Stonehocker J. Barriers to intrauterine device insertion in postpartum women. Contraception 2005;72(6):426–9.
5. Global Health Observatory (GHO) Data. World Health Organization; 2015. Available at: http://www.who.int/gho/health_workforce/nursing_midwifery_density/en/. Accessed May 11, 2015.
6. Weston MR, Martins SL, Neustadt AB, et al. Factors influencing uptake of intrauterine devices among postpartum adolescents: a qualitative study. Am J Obstet Gynecol 2012;206(1):40.e1–7.
7. Asker C, Stokes-Lampard H, Beavan J, et al. What is it about intrauterine devices that women find unacceptable? Factors that make women non-users: a qualitative study. J Fam Plann Reprod Health Care 2006;32(2):89–94.
8. Hubacher D, Reyes V, Lillo S, et al. Pain from copper intrauterine device insertion: randomized trial of prophylactic ibuprofen. Am J Obstet Gynecol 2006;195(5): 1272–7.
9. Goldstuck ND, Matthews ML. A comparison of the actual and expected pain response following insertion of an intrauterine contraceptive device. Clin Reprod Fertil 1985;3(1):65–71.
10. Murty J. Use and effectiveness of oral analgesia when fitting an intrauterine device. J Fam Plann Reprod Health Care 2003;29(3):150–1.
11. Bednarek PH, Creinin MD, Reeves MF, et al. Prophylactic ibuprofen does not improve pain with IUD insertion: a randomized trial. Contraception 2015;91(3): 193–7.
12. Chen BA, Reeves MF, Hayes JL, et al. Postplacental or delayed insertion of the levonorgestrel intrauterine device after vaginal delivery: a randomized controlled trial. Obstet Gynecol 2010;116(5):1079–87.
13. Xu JX, Rivera R, Dunson TR, et al. A comparative study of two techniques used in immediate postplacental insertion (IPPI) of the Copper T-380A IUD in Shanghai, People's Republic of China. Contraception 1996;54(1):33–8.
14. Committee on Adolescent Health Care Long-Acting Reversible Contraception Working Group, The American College of Obstetricians and Gynecologists.

Committee opinion no. 539: adolescents and long-acting reversible contraception: implants and intrauterine devices. Obstet Gynecol 2012;120(4):983–8.

15. Prager S, Darney PD. The levonorgestrel intrauterine system in nulliparous women. Contraception 2007;75(6 Suppl):S12–5.

16. Madden T, McNicholas C, Zhao Q, et al. Association of age and parity with intrauterine device expulsion. Obstet Gynecol 2014;124(4):718–26.

17. Kapp N, Curtis KM. Intrauterine device insertion during the postpartum period: a systematic review. Contraception 2009;80(4):327–36.

18. Lester F, Kakaire O, Byamugisha J, et al. Intracesarean insertion of the Copper T380A versus 6 weeks postcesarean: a randomized clinical trial. Contraception 2015;91(3):198–203.

19. Celen S, Moroy P, Sucak A, et al. Clinical outcomes of early postplacental insertion of intrauterine contraceptive devices. Contraception 2004;69(4):279–82.

20. Chi IC, Wilkens L, Rogers S. Expulsions in immediate postpartum insertions of Lippes Loop D and Copper T IUDs and their counterpart Delta devices–an epidemiological analysis. Contraception 1985;32(2):119–34.

21. Grimes DA, Lopez LM, Schulz KF, et al. Immediate post-partum insertion of intrauterine devices. Cochrane Database Syst Rev 2010;(5):CD003036.

22. Heinemann K, Reed S, Moehner S, et al. Risk of uterine perforation with levonorgestrel-releasing and copper intrauterine devices in the European Active Surveillance Study on Intrauterine Devices. Contraception 2015;91(4):274–9.

23. Centers for Disease Control and Prevention. US Medical Eligibility Criteria for Contraception Use, 2010: Adapted from the World Health Organization Medical Eligibility Criteria for Contraceptive Use, 4th edition. MMWR 2010;59(No. RR-4):1-88.

24. Washington CI, Jamshidi R, Thung SF, et al. Timing of postpartum intrauterine device placement: a cost-effectiveness analysis. Fertil Steril 2015;103(1):131–7.

Immediate Intrauterine Device Insertion Following Surgical Abortion

Eva Patil, MD, Paula H. Bednarek, MD, MPH*

KEYWORDS

- Intrauterine device • Postabortion intrauterine device insertion
- Postaspiration intrauterine device insertion
- Postdilation and evacuation intrauterine device • Contraception

KEY POINTS

- Intrauterine device (IUD) insertion is safe immediately after a first trimester aspiration procedure for abortion or miscarriage management.
- IUD insertion is safe immediately after a second trimester dilation and evacuation procedure.
- Risk of IUD expulsion increases slightly with increasing uterine size at time of placement.
- Providing women with immediate highly effective contraception is convenient, increases contraception continuation, and decreases unintended pregnancy.

BACKGROUND

In the United States, approximately 50% of the 6 million pregnancies that occur each year are unintended, and half of these end in abortion.[1] About one-half of abortions occur in women who have had a previous abortion.[2] Consequently, contraceptive counseling and the option of immediate initiation of effective contraception are critical components of abortion care. Immediate initiation of any contraceptive method following abortion results in a lower risk of repeat abortion, with immediate insertion of an intrauterine device (IUD) being most effective in reducing this risk.[3,4] IUD placement immediately after abortion eliminates the need for an additional visit to obtain highly effective contraception prior to the next ovulation, which can occur as early

Disclosure Statement: Dr E. Patil has no disclosures. Dr P.H. Bednarek has served on an Advisory Board for Bayer.
Department of Obstetrics and Gynecology, Oregon Health & Science University, 3181 Southwest Sam Jackson Park Road, Mail code UHN50, Portland, OR 97239, USA
* Corresponding author.
E-mail address: bednarek@ohsu.edu

as 2 to 3 weeks after the procedure.[5] Mathematical modeling has estimated that moving from delayed IUD insertion to insertion immediately following abortion would prevent over 70,000 unintended pregnancies annually in the United States.[6]

CONTINUATION AND EXPULSION

Many women who intend to use an IUD for contraception following abortion do not follow-up after the procedure and thus do not receive interval IUD placement.[7–10] In a randomized controlled trial of 88 women undergoing dilation and evacuation (D&E) receiving either immediate or delayed (3–6 weeks after the procedure) levonorgestrel-releasing IUD, only 45.5% of the delayed insertion subjects returned for IUD placement compared with 100% of women who received their IUD in the immediate insertion group.[11] Additionally, of the subjects who were contacted by phone 6 months after the abortion, only 17 of 27 (62.9%) were using the IUD in the delayed insertion group compared with 23 of 27 (85.2%) in the immediate insertion group.[11] In another study, 215 women undergoing second trimester D&E were randomized to immediate versus delayed placement of a copper T380 A IUD. Of 104 subjects randomized to receive immediate postabortion IUD placement, 71 could be reached by phone after 6 months, and 81.7% (58 of 71) of women were still using the IUD for contraception. IUD use with immediate postabortion placement was significantly higher than the group in which IUD placement was delayed 2 to 4 weeks after the procedure. Of the 111 women randomized to this group, 88 could be reached, and 28.4% (25/88) were using an IUD after 6 months ($P = .003$).[12] No patients who received immediate IUD insertion had a repeat pregnancy at 6 months compared with 8.4% in the delayed group ($P = .022$).[12] These studies reinforce the importance of weighing the increased risk of expulsion against the risk of repeat unplanned pregnancy.

The risk of IUD expulsion appears to be higher with immediate postabortion placement compared with interval placement, although reported expulsion rates in studies vary.[7–11,13] For interval IUD placement, expulsion risk is most commonly estimated to be 5%, although studies report anywhere between a 2% and 10% expulsion rate.[14] A randomized trial of parous women receiving interval placement of either a levonorgestrel or copper IUD demonstrated an expulsion rate of 6.3 and 5.6 per 100 women respectively in the first year of use.[15] Placement after first or second trimester surgical abortion has been shown to be a risk factor for expulsion.[9] Risk of expulsion after first trimester aspiration abortion is reported between 0.8 % and 7%[8,10,13] and between 3% and 8% after second trimester D&E.[8,11,13] The difference in expulsion risk between placement after first or second trimester procedures in these studies was often not statistically different, although studies were not adequately powered to detect differences in this outcome. Although the risk of IUD expulsion may be higher with postabortion placement, the provision of this highly effective contraceptive immediately after abortion outweighs the increased risk of expulsion for most women who request this option.

PREPROCEDURE PREPARATION
Sexually Transmitted Infection Screening

If a woman has not been screened for sexually transmitted infections (STIs) according the US Centers for Disease Control (CDC) or US Preventive Services Task Force (USPSTF) recommendations, then screening can be performed at the start of the abortion procedure. Both the CDC and USPSTF recommend screening for *Chlamydia trachomatis* at least once per year in all sexually active women younger than 25 years of age, as well as older women who have risk factors for STI acquisition (eg, a new partner or more than 1 sexual partner).[16,17] Many clinicians choose to screen for *Neisseria gonorrhea* and *C trachomatis* in all women prior to IUD insertion, although this practice is not based on any data or national guidelines. Randomized controlled trials have not shown any correlation between *Chlamydia*-positive screening prior to the abortion procedure and pelvic infection afterward.[10,13]

After the tests have been collected, there is no need to wait for results prior to the abortion or IUD insertion. If a woman is found to have gonorrhea or chlamydia, she and her partner(s) should be treated with appropriate antibiotics, but the IUD does not need to be removed.[18]

Antibiotic Prophylaxis

Both the American Congress of Obstetrics and Gynecology (ACOG) and the Society of Family Planning (SFP) support perioperative antibiotics in women undergoing first and second trimester surgical abortion.[19,20] A meta-analysis by Sawaya and colleagues[21] included 12 randomized controlled trials that demonstrated a 42% reduction in postabortal infections in women given periprocedural antibiotics compared with those who were not. Studies evaluating immediate postabortion IUD insertion reported no difference in rates of uterine infection between patients who received an immediate postabortion IUD versus those who had an abortion alone.[9,10] Therefore, routine perioperative antibiotics for the abortion are recommended, but no additional antibiotics are recommended if an IUD will be placed at that time.[20]

Abortion Complications

Complications following surgical abortion are rare, but if hemorrhage, uterine perforation, or hematometra occurs, the IUD should generally not be placed immediately following the surgical abortion. An IUD should not be placed in the setting of a septic abortion. Women should be offered an interim contraceptive method, and they can return for IUD insertion after the complication has resolved.

INTRAUTERINE DEVICE INSERTION AFTER FIRST TRIMESTER SURGICAL ABORTION

Published in the first trimester data do not suggest an optimal technique for immediate postabortion IUD insertion. Here are described techniques used by experienced providers. When placing an IUD immediately after surgical abortion, bimanual examination and evaluation of the cervix will have already been done. Providers should confirm no complications have occurred; bleeding is minimal, and the abortion is complete by examining the products of conception, using ultrasound, or both. Some providers may choose to recleanse the cervix with povidone iodine or betadine.

Sounding (Assessing Uterine Size)

It is important to assess uterine cavity size immediately before placing the IUD. The uterus contracts quickly following completion of the abortion, and may be smaller for IUD insertion than during the abortion procedure. Many clinicians use the cannula that was used for the abortion as a sound, because it has a broad tip and is readily available. Alternatives would be to use a dilator or the IUD inserter itself. Generally, the typical narrow uterine sound is avoided, because a larger instrument can pass through the cervix and a theoretic concern for an increased risk of perforation has been suggested.

Intrauterine Device Placement Technique

After first trimester abortion, most clinicians use the standard technique with the manufacturer-provided inserter.[13] **Fig. 1** lists instructions. Occasionally, the inserter

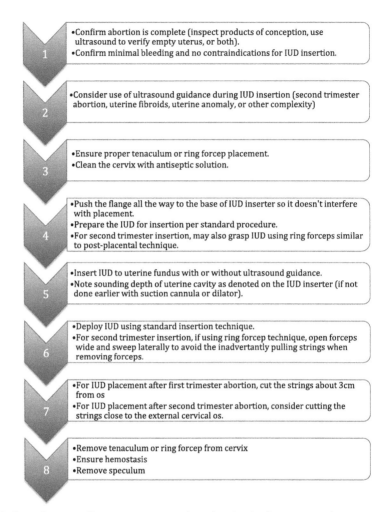

Fig. 1. Steps for immediate IUD insertion after abortion in first or second trimester.

may need to be grasped with a sterile ring forceps to guide it past irregularities in the uterine contour to reach the desired placement at the fundus. The strings are generally cut to about 3 cm, similar to interval insertion.

INTRAUTERINE DEVICE INSERTION IMMEDIATELY AFTER SECOND TRIMESTER SURGICAL ABORTION

Women undergoing second trimester abortion with either dilation and evacuation (D&E) or other techniques should be offered a full range of contraceptive options. Often women in need of second trimester abortion are among the most vulnerable populations, including adolescents, women experiencing disruptive life events including financial hardships, members of minority groups, and women who are underinsured and less educated.[22,23] These women can benefit from long-acting, highly effective contraceptive methods, and the option of immediate placement of an IUD is highly desirable.

Women with health conditions or fetal complications also seek second trimester abortion. Physicians may incorrectly assume women who terminate a pregnancy because of a fetal complication prefer immediate postprocedure attempts at conception. Although some women may desire pregnancy, others will prefer to use contraception. Women with health conditions may need an opportunity to optimize conditions such as hypertension or diabetes, or they may desire time to grieve the loss of the current pregnancy. In these cases, an IUD is an excellent contraceptive option. Providers should address contraception with every woman seeking D&E for any indication.

Intrauterine Device Placement Technique

Immediate postabortion IUD placement in the second trimester is similar to placement in the first trimester, with a few key exceptions. The size of the uterine cavity can be determined by the depth of the suction cannula at the time of abortion completion or with the IUD inserter itself. Frequently the IUD inserter can be used in the same manner as in interval placement. Occasionally, placement with a ring forceps or with a sterile gloved hand is needed if the inserter is not long enough, or if there are uterine irregularities, such as intracavitary fibroids.[13,24] This can be done in a similar fashion to postplacental IUD placement (see images and technique details in the article concerning postpartum).

ULTRASOUND GUIDANCE

Many experienced providers recommend using ultrasound guidance for immediate postabortion in the first trimester IUD insertion, although no studies have evaluated whether this practice routinely is beneficial. Ultrasound guidance during insertion can be helpful for women with uterine anomalies like fibroids or a particularly flexed uterus to ensure fundal placement of the device. If ultrasound was not used during the insertion, then ultrasound performed immediately after IUD placement may help to confirm IUD location.[10] This may be useful in training settings.

Ultrasound during second trimester D&E has been shown to decrease complications, specifically in training institutions.[25] Although there has not been any study specifically studying ultrasound guidance with immediate postabortion IUD insertion, this practice is advocated by many experienced providers. The contours of the uterine cavity can make fundal placement challenging, and visual confirmation by ultrasound can ensure the fundal placement of the device.

Early evaluations of immediate IUD insertion following second trimester abortion revealed unacceptably high rates of expulsion by 120 days when comparing 3 devices no longer used in the United States (19.5% for TCU220C, 48.8% for Lippes Loop and 21.3% for Cooper 7).[26] However, routine use of ultrasound guidance for immediate IUD placement appears to help ensure fundal placement and with lower expulsion risks (1%–3% after first trimester D&C and 3%–7% after second trimester D&E).[8,13] Ultrasound guidance has become common practice in the United States for immediate IUD insertion following second trimester abortion to ensure fundal IUD placement.[8,24]

BLEEDING PATTERNS

Limited data on bleeding patterns following immediate postabortion IUD insertion suggest IUD insertion does not significantly alter postabortion bleeding patterns. Subanalysis of a large randomized controlled trial comparing immediate with delayed IUD insertion following first trimester abortion showed that immediate IUD does not increase bleeding or spotting during the first 28 days after aspiration.[27] Cramping that requires pain medication is slightly increased during the first 14 days following immediate postabortion IUD insertion, but is no different thereafter.

There also has been a published subanalysis of a trial that compared bleeding patterns among women who had either a copper or a levonorgestrel IUD placed immediately after abortion or 3 to 10 days after the onset of menses.[28] The timing of insertion was not randomized, but choice of IUD was randomized. Women with postabortion IUD insertion had slightly better bleeding patterns than those with postmenstrual insertion. The bleeding patterns appeared to be established during the first few months with little change thereafter.

FOLLOW-UP

Expected changes in bleeding and warning signs of infection or expulsion should be reviewed with all patients after insertion. A follow-up visit can provide an opportunity for additional counseling regarding changes in bleeding or other concerns that might result in premature removal of the device. However, a routine follow-up visit is not necessary for all patients and can be individualized. If there is concern for expulsion or IUD perforation, a woman may feel for her IUD strings. If not able to feel the strings, she should then be instructed to use a backup contraceptive method and return for evaluation. Regardless, women should be encouraged to return at any time if they have concerns or questions.[18]

SAFETY AND COMPLICATIONS

Extensive data show that immediate IUD insertion following first or second trimester abortion is safe.[9] Rates of infection, perforation, retained products of conception, and need for reaspiration are low and have not been found to be significantly different if IUD placement is added to the abortion procedure.[8,9,11,13] Both progestin and copper IUDs have been used immediately after first and second trimester surgical abortions. Postabortion IUD insertion studies have not included Skyla; however, no data suggest Skyla would have a different safety profile when inserted after abortion. The World Health Organization (WHO) Medical Eligibility Criteria and US Medical Eligibility Criteria for Contraceptive Use both list the placement of an IUD immediately following first trimester abortion as a category 1, or no restriction.[26,29]

Perforation

IUD perforation is a rare, but recognized potential complication of IUD use. It is estimated to occur at a frequency of 0 to 1.3 cases per 1000 interval insertions.[30] Data show no evidence of a different perforation risk with immediate postabortion IUD placement compared with interval insertion. A multicenter randomized trial that followed 578 women for 6 months reported no IUD perforations. However, 1 perforation during the aspiration procedure was noted, and that subject was deemed ineligible for immediate IUD insertion.[10] Anecdotally, many experienced providers suggest perforation is less likely when an IUD is inserted immediately following surgical abortion, because the dilated cervix provides no resistance to the passage of the IUD. If perforation is not recognized during placement but suspected at a follow-up visit, the location of the IUD should be verified. This is done by checking for appropriate length strings visible at the cervix. If strings are not seen, an ultrasound should be performed. If no intrauterine IUD is identified, an abdominal radiograph can identify if an IUD is intraperitoneal, which is typically removed laparoscopically.

Delayed Complications

Patients who have an IUD placed following a first or second trimester abortion may encounter the same complications as other abortion patients, but pain, irregular or heavy bleeding, or infection are unlikely to be specifically caused by the IUD. For this reason, it is usually not necessary or helpful to remove the IUD while these complications are being evaluated and treated. An IUD does not need to be removed in the setting of endometritis unless the patient does not show clinical improvement with the use of antibiotics.[31,32]

PATIENT EXPERIENCE

Returning to the clinic for follow-up after an abortion is challenging for many women. Many women travel significant distances for abortion care. Some women wish to maintain privacy surrounding the abortion and decline follow-up. Satisfaction following immediate postabortion IUD placement appears to be high, although studies have been limited by low follow-up rates. In a retrospective study of 77 women who had undergone immediate postabortion IUD insertion following both first and second trimester abortion, satisfaction and continuation were both 80% at a mean follow-up time of 9 months. In a retrospective study of 123 women who received an immediate IUD insertion after first trimester abortion and 133 after second trimester abortion who were not lost to follow-up, 94% were satisfied with their IUD 6 or more weeks after insertion.[13]

Another study of 121 women who received immediate IUD after surgical abortion at a mean gestation age of 14.2 weeks found 93% were satisfied with their IUD at the time of phone follow-up around 8 weeks after the procedure.[33] However, this study also found that 16% of these women had questions about their bleeding pattern; 15% had questions about pain or cramping symptoms, and 10% had questions about string management.[33] Overall, patients are highly satisfied with immediate IUD insertion following surgical abortion and have high continuation rates. However, study findings highlight the importance of patient counseling about expected symptoms following IUD placement.

SUMMARY

Effective contraceptive services are integral to the care of patients undergoing abortion. A woman's short- and long-term reproductive plans should be discussed to help guide her choice of contraceptive method to best meet her needs. Assuming no immediate complications, it is safe to place an IUD immediately following surgical abortion in the first or second trimester. Given that IUDs are highly effective at preventing repeat unintended pregnancy, if a patient desires an IUD, immediate placement is recommended as a best practice following first or second trimester abortion.

REFERENCES

1. Finer LB, Henshaw SK. Disparities in rates of unintended pregnancy in the United States, 1994 and 2001. Perspect Sex Reprod Health 2006;38(2):90–6.
2. Jones RK, Darroch JE, Henshaw SK. Contraceptive use among U.S. women having abortions in 2000-2001. Perspect Sex Reprod Health 2002;34(6):294–303.
3. Heikinheimo O, Gissler M, Suhonen S. Age, parity, history of abortion and contraceptive choices affect the risk of repeat abortion. Contraception 2008;78(2): 149–54.

4. Goodman S, Hendlish SK, Reeves MF, et al. Impact of immediate postabortal insertion of intrauterine contraception on repeat abortion. Contraception 2008; 78(2):143–8.

5. Marrs RP, Kletzky OA, Howard WF, et al. Disappearance of human chorionic gonadotropin and resumption of ovulation following abortion. Am J Obstet Gynecol 1979;135(6):731–6.

6. Reeves MF, Smith KJ, Creinin MD. Contraceptive effectiveness of immediate compared with delayed insertion of intrauterine devices after abortion: a decision analysis. Obstet Gynecol 2007;109(6):1286–94.

7. Stanwood NL, Grimes DA, Schulz KF. Insertion of an intrauterine contraceptive device after induced or spontaneous abortion: a review of the evidence. BJOG Int J Obstet Gynaecol 2001;108(11):1168–73.

8. Fox MC, Oat-Judge J, Severson K, et al. Immediate placement of intrauterine devices after first and second trimester pregnancy termination. Contraception 2011; 83(1):34–40.

9. Okusanya BO, Oduwole O, Effa EE. Immediate postabortal insertion of intrauterine devices. Cochrane Database Syst Rev 2014;(7):CD001777.

10. Bednarek PH, Creinin MD, Reeves MF, et al. Immediate versus delayed IUD insertion after uterine aspiration. N Engl J Med 2011;364(23):2208–17.

11. Hohmann HL, Reeves MF, Chen BA, et al. Immediate versus delayed insertion of the levonorgestrel-releasing intrauterine device following dilation and evacuation: a randomized controlled trial. Contraception 2012;85(3):240–5.

12. Cremer M, Bullard KA, Mosley RM, et al. Immediate vs. delayed post-abortal copper T 380A IUD insertion in cases over 12 weeks of gestation. Contraception 2011;83(6):522–7.

13. Drey EA, Reeves MF, Ogawa DD, et al. Insertion of intrauterine contraceptives immediately following first- and second-trimester abortions. Contraception 2009;79(5):397–402.

14. Madden T, McNicholas C, Zhao Q, et al. Association of age and parity with intrauterine device expulsion. Obstet Gynecol 2014;124(4):718–26.

15. Sivin I, el Mahgoub S, McCarthy T, et al. Long-term contraception with the levonorgestrel 20 mcg/day (LNg 20) and the copper T 380Ag intrauterine devices: a five-year randomized study. Contraception 1990;42(4):361–78.

16. Workowski KA, Berman S, Centers for Disease Control and Prevention (CDC). 2010 STD treatment guidelines. MMWR Recomm Rep 2010;59:1–110. Available at: http://www.cdc.gov/std/treatment/2010/. Accessed May 14, 2015.

17. LeFevre ML. Screening for Chlamydia and Gonorrhea: U.S. Preventive Services Task Force Recommendation Statement Screening for Chlamydia and Gonorrhea. Ann Intern Med 2014;161(12):902–10.

18. Centers for Disease Control and Prevention (CDC). U.S. selected practice recommendations for contraceptive use. MMWR Recomm Rep 2013;62(RR05): 1–46.

19. The American College of Obstetricians and Gynecologists. Practice bulletin: second trimester abortion. June 2013.

20. Achilles SL, Reeves MF. Prevention of infection after induced abortion. Contraception 2011;83(4):295–309.

21. Sawaya GF, Grady D, Kerlikowske K, et al. Antibiotics at the time of induced abortion: the case for universal prophylaxis based on a meta-analysis. Obstet Gynecol 1996;87(5 Part 2):884–90.

22. Jones RK, Finer LB. Who has second-trimester abortions in the United States? Contraception 2012;85(6):544–51.

23. Drey EA, Foster DG, Jackson RA, et al. Risk factors associated with presenting for abortion in the second trimester. Obstet Gynecol 2006;107(1):128–35.
24. Paul M, Lichtenberg ES, Borgatta L, et al. Management of unintended and abnormal pregnancy: comprehensive abortion care. Chichester (United Kingdom): Wiley-Blackwell; 2009.
25. Darney PD, Sweet RL. Routine intraoperative ultrasonography for second trimester abortion reduces incidence of uterine perforation. J Ultrasound Med 1989;8(2):71–5.
26. Department of Reproductive Health. WHO | Medical eligibility criteria for contraceptive use, 4th edition. 2010. Available at: http://www.who.int/reproductivehealth/publications/family_planning/9789241563888/en/. Accessed May 14, 2015.
27. Bednarek PH, Botha RL, Creinin MD, et al. The effect of immediate intrauterine device (IUD) insertion on bleeding patterns following first trimester suction aspiration. Fertil Steril 2009;92(3 Supplement):S27.
28. Suvisaari J, Lähteenmäki P. Detailed analysis of menstrual bleeding patterns after postmenstrual and postabortal insertion of a copper IUD or a levonorgestrel-releasing intrauterine system. Contraception 1996;54(4):201–8.
29. Update to CDC's U.S. Medical eligibility criteria for contraceptive use, 2010: revised recommendations for the use of contraceptive methods during the postpartum period. Available at: http://www.cdc.gov/mmwr/preview/mmwrhtml/mm6026a3.htm. Accessed July 22, 2014.
30. Andersson K, Ryde-Blomqvist E, Lindell K, et al. Perforations with intrauterine devices: Report from a Swedish survey. Contraception 1998;57(4):251–5.
31. Rinehart W. WHO updates medical eligibility criteria for contraceptives. Baltimore (MD): Johns Hopkins University; 2004.
32. Improving access to quality care in family planning: medical eligibility criteria for contraceptive use. 3rd edition. Geneva (Switzerland): World Health Organization; 2003.
33. Diedrich JT, Drey EA, Dehlendorf C, et al. Women's questions after postabortion insertion of intrauterine contraception. Contraception 2013;88(3):396–400.

Therapeutic Options for Unscheduled Bleeding Associated with Long-Acting Reversible Contraception

EmmaKate Friedlander, MD*, Bliss Kaneshiro, MD, MPH

KEYWORDS

- Irregular bleeding • Intrauterine device • Contraceptive implant • Levonorgestrel
- Etonogestrel

KEY POINTS

- Long-acting reversible contraception (LARCs), including intrauterine devices and implants, are highly effective forms of birth control.
- Irregular vaginal bleeding is one of the most common reasons for premature discontinuation of LARC devices.
- Nonsteroidal antiinflammatory drugs can decrease unscheduled bleeding associated with LARC use and are the most well studied for this indication.
- Other medications that can decrease unscheduled bleeding include antifibrinolytics (tranexamic acid), antiprogestins (mifepristone), and matrix metalloproteinase inhibitors (doxycycline).

INTRODUCTION

Long-acting reversible contraception (LARC), such as intrauterine devices (IUDs) and implants, are the most effective reversible contraceptives available.[1] A common side effect of both IUDs and implants is an alteration in menstrual bleeding patterns. Women can experience heavier bleeding with the copper IUD or unscheduled bleeding and spotting with the hormonal and copper IUD as well as the contraceptive implant. Dissatisfaction with bleeding, particularly heavy or unscheduled bleeding and spotting, is a common reason for early discontinuation of LARC methods.[2] Therapies that can prevent or treat unscheduled bleeding could improve patient satisfaction, increase uptake of LARC methods, and reduce early discontinuation, all of which would result in fewer unplanned pregnancies.

Family Planning Division, Department of Obstetrics, Gynecology and Women's Health, University of Hawaii John A. Burns School of Medicine, 1319 Punahou Street, #824, Honolulu, HI 96826, USA
* Corresponding author.
E-mail address: emmakate@hawaii.edu

Obstet Gynecol Clin N Am 42 (2015) 593–603
http://dx.doi.org/10.1016/j.ogc.2015.07.004
0889-8545/15/$ – see front matter © 2015 Elsevier Inc. All rights reserved.

obgyn.theclinics.com

The reason women experience unscheduled bleeding with IUDs and implants has not been clearly elucidated. Unscheduled bleeding falls into 2 categories: bleeding that occurs with initiation of a LARC method and bleeding that occurs with prolonged use of LARC. Bleeding that occurs with initiation of a levonorgestrel (LNG) IUD and etonogestrel (ENG) implant is common and is most likely the result of the endometrium transitioning to a thin state from consistent progestin exposure. The precise mechanism of unscheduled bleeding that occurs with prolonged exposure to progestin is unknown but is thought to be related to the progestin dilating superficial veins and capillaries, which are fragile and susceptible to focal bleeding. Other potential influences include changes in structural support in the endometrium, altered matrix metalloproteinase (MMP) activity, and changes in endometrial perfusion and hemostasis.

Structured direct counseling before LARC initiation to inform women about common bleeding patterns associated with each contraceptive method is critical to method initiation and acceptance. Emphasizing that unscheduled bleeding is not associated with decreased efficacy of the method is key. Advance knowledge of possible unscheduled bleeding may reassure users, that if bleeding irregularities occur, the method is still effective; users may be willing to wait longer for unscheduled bleeding or spotting to resolve.

Pregnancy should always be excluded first when new-onset amenorrhea is accompanied by signs or symptoms of pregnancy. If a woman with an IUD complains of both irregular bleeding and pelvic pain, it is important to verify proper placement by examination or ultrasound to ensure that the device is not in the cervix, embedded in the myometrium, or perforated through the uterus. Consideration should also be given to infections or pathologic causes like cervical or endometrial cancer. Cultures or endometrial biopsies can be done with an IUD in place.

Heavy, prolonged, and unscheduled bleeding are strongly associated with dissatisfaction and early discontinuation of LARC methods.[3–6] Clinicians must, therefore, be armed with evidence-based interventions to alleviate this common side effect. The authors review the current literature related to the treatment of unscheduled bleeding and spotting that accompanies IUD and contraceptive implant use, discuss major themes in the treatment of unscheduled bleeding, and identify areas where further research is needed. In the authors' review of the literature, they limited their search to human subjects and articles published in English. The authors excluded treatment modalities that are not available in the United States.

COPPER INTRAUTERINE DEVICE

With the copper IUD (copper T380A/Paragard [Teva Women's Health, Inc, Sellersville, PA, USA]), irregular spotting and prolonged or heavier menses are frequent in the first few months of use. Menstrual bleeding can be increased up to 55% to 74%, which is thought to be because of excessive prostaglandin release in the endometrial cavity.[7,8] The discontinuation rate for pain or bleeding in one trial of the copper T380A was 5% at 1 year, 8% at 2 years, and 9% at 3 years.[9]

Interventions for Heavy Bleeding

Treatments for heavy bleeding associated with copper IUD use include nonsteroidal antiinflammatory drugs (NSAIDs), antifibrinolytic agents, and antidiuretics. Some trials have also studied prophylactic interventions to prevent the initial increase in bleeding known to occur for most users. **Table 1** contains a summary of medical interventions shown to have a benefit in clinical trials for heavy bleeding in copper IUD users.

Table 1
Medical interventions for heavy bleeding in copper IUD users

Timing	Medication Class	Medication	Dose	Frequency	Length of Time
Prophylaxis	NSAID	Ibuprofen	400 mg	3 Times daily	10 d
	Antifibrinolytic	Tranexamic acid	500 mg	2 Times daily	5 d
		Tranexamic acid	1000 mg	2 Times daily	5 d
Treatment	NSAID	Ibuprofen	400 mg	4 Times daily	7 d
		Indomethacin	25 mg	2 Times daily	7 d
		Indomethacin	25 mg	4 Times daily	3 d
		Mefenamic acid	100 mg	3 Times daily	3 d
		Mefenamic acid	500 mg	3 Times daily	5 d
		Diclofenac	50 mg	3 Times daily	1 d, then
			25 mg	3 Times daily	4 d
	Antifibrinolytic	Tranexamic acid	1500 mg	3 Times daily	5 d
	Antidiuretic	Desmopressin	300 mcg	Intranasal daily	5 d

Nonsteroidal antiinflammatory drugs

NSAIDs such as ibuprofen, indomethacin, mefenamic acid, and diclofenac are the most widely studied for blood loss reduction in copper IUD users. NSAIDs inhibit prostaglandin synthesis and decrease endometrial prostaglandin release.

Exploring NSAIDs as a prophylactic measure, ibuprofen 400 mg was administered 3 times daily for 10 days with the first menses after IUD insertion in a randomized controlled trial of 28 new copper IUD users with previously normal menses. Women who received prophylactic ibuprofen had less menstrual blood loss compared with women who received placebo ($P<.05$). When compared with preinsertion values, blood loss increased by 74% in the placebo group and 2% in the ibuprofen group ($P<.01$).[7] This trial did not collect data on menses after stopping the intervention, so it is unclear if the prophylactic treatment had a sustained effect or if benefits were limited to the first cycle. Taking a prolonged course of ibuprofen with each menstrual period may be impractical for many women.

As a treatment of heavy bleeding, ibuprofen 400 mg 4 times daily for 7 days initiated on the first day of menses in copper IUD users decreased blood loss by 25% in one trial ($P<.05$).[10] Indomethacin 25 mg 4 times daily for 3 days with menses was also associated with a significant reduction in blood loss of 38% ($P<.01$).[11] Another trial of indomethacin used 25 mg twice daily for 7 days initiated at the start of menses in women who reported heavy or prolonged bleeding and noted a significant reduction in the number of bleeding/spotting days (10 fewer days per 90-day cycle) as well as length of bleeding episode (approximately 3 days less).[12] Mefenamic acid 100 mg 3 times daily for 3 days, given several days before expected menstruation or with the start of menses, was also associated with a significant reduction in blood loss ($P<.01$).[13] Higher doses of mefenamic acid, 500 mg 3 times daily for 5 days starting with menses, were associated with a reduction in mean blood loss of 47.5% ($P<.001$).[14] Diclofenac sodium 50 mg 3 times daily for 1 day, followed by 25 mg 3 times daily for 4 days decreased mean blood loss by 20%, though no change was seen in pelvic pain or duration of menses.[15]

Aspirin is not recommended as a treatment of unscheduled bleeding. In one trial, aspirin 1000 mg 3 times daily for 5 days starting with menses in women with a copper IUD resulted in significantly increased menstrual bleeding in women whose baseline mean blood loss was less than 60 mL ($P<.05$). Treatment was not associated with significant changes in blood loss in women with a baseline mean blood loss of 60 to 80 mL or more than 80 mL.[16]

Antifibrinolytic agents

Antifibrinolytic agents, such as tranexamic acid, are thought to reduce heavy bleeding by preventing the degradation of fibrin. Lin and colleagues[17] compared bleeding with first menses after copper IUD insertion when participants took prophylactic tranexamic acid 500 mg or 1000 mg twice daily for 5 days versus placebo. All groups had an increase in blood loss in the first cycle, which then decreased over subsequent cycles. Both doses of tranexamic acid were associated with significantly less blood loss (approximately 20 mL less) compared with placebo (P<.05). The higher dose of tranexamic acid did not confer an additional benefit. Both tranexamic acid groups also had significantly fewer participants with blood loss of more than 80 mL per cycle compared with placebo. In another trial of therapeutic tranexamic acid, 1500 mg 3 times daily for 5 days with menses significantly decreased menstrual blood loss by 54% (P<.001), though a change in pelvic pain intensity or duration of menses was not noted.[15]

Antidiuretics

Antidiuretics like desmopressin, a synthetic version of vasopressin, are theorized to decrease heavy bleeding by acting as a vasoconstrictor. Desmopressin 300 mcg intranasal daily for 5 days with menses led to a significant reduction in blood loss of 40.5% in a trial of women with menorrhagia associated with a copper IUD.[14]

Summary of Recommendations for Heavy Bleeding with the Copper Intrauterine Device

For prophylaxis against heavy bleeding in new copper IUD users, consider ibuprofen or tranexamic acid starting with the first day of menses. For treatment of heavy bleeding once a copper IUD is in place, consider NSAIDs first, including ibuprofen, indomethacin, mefenamic acid, and diclofenac, each started on the first day of menses. Other promising interventions to treat heavy bleeding associated with the copper IUD include tranexamic acid and desmopressin. Aspirin is not recommended.

LEVONORGESTREL INTRAUTERINE DEVICE

Overall, progestin-containing IUDs are associated with decreased menstrual bleeding or amenorrhea. After 6 months, 44% of women using the LNG 20 (Mirena [Bayer HealthCare Pharmaceuticals Inc, Wayne, NJ, USA]) (releases 20 mcg of LNG per day) reported amenorrhea. This proportion increased to 50% after 12 and 24 months of use.[18] Increased intermenstrual bleeding and spotting are also commonly noted with LNG 20 IUD use. Thirty-five percent of users experience frequent or prolonged bleeding, defined as more than 4 episodes of bleeding in 90 days or one episode lasting more than 10 days, in the first 3 months of use. This proportion decreases to 4% by 1 year of use.[8] The likelihood of improved bleeding over time is encouraging, yet the discontinuation rate for menstrual disturbance is 5.9% and is the most frequently cited reason for discontinuation.[4]

Similar bleeding patterns are seen with the LNG 14 IUD (Skyla) (releases 14 mcg of LNG per day), though amenorrhea is less common. Unscheduled bleeding is common in the first 3 months of use, with 59% of women reporting prolonged bleeding, 42% reporting irregular bleeding, and 31% reporting frequent bleeding. These proportions decrease to 9%, 23%, and 8%, respectively, at the end of 1 year. At 1 year, 6% of women report amenorrhea, increasing to 12% at year 3. The discontinuation rate for menstrual disturbance with the LNG 14 IUD is approximately 5%.[3]

Comprehensive structured counseling before LNG IUD insertion and reassurance when unscheduled bleeding occurs is integral to a clinical practice that includes IUD insertion. Historically, clinicians prescribed cyclic combined oral contraceptive pills in addition to the IUD if bothersome unscheduled bleeding occurred. This prescription provided endometrial stabilization with estrogen while maintaining the superior contraceptive efficacy of the IUD. Although this was shown to be beneficial in levonorgestrel implant (Norplant) users, no data currently support this practice with the LNG IUD.

Treatment of Irregular Bleeding

Similar to copper IUD trials, interventions for irregular bleeding associated with the LNG 20 IUD include NSAIDs (naproxen and mefenamic acid) and antifibrinolytic agents (tranexamic acid). Other interventions studied include estrogen, antiprogestins (mifepristone), and selective progesterone receptor modulators (SPRMs; like ulipristal acetate). No interventions to decrease irregular bleeding with the LNG 14 IUD have been studied to date. **Table 2** contains a summary of medical interventions shown to have a benefit in clinical trials for irregular bleeding in LNG IUD users.

Nonsteroidal antiinflammatory drugs

Naproxen 500 mg twice daily for 5 days, beginning the day after LNG 20 insertion and repeated monthly for 3 cycles, was associated with a 10% decrease in bleeding and spotting days. When the number of bleeding and spotting days were divided into quartiles, the naproxen group was most likely to be in the lowest quartile when compared with placebo (42.9% vs 16.3%; $P = .03$). However, 4 weeks after treatment, the effects did not persist; no difference in bleeding or spotting days was noted.[19]

Mefenamic acid 500 mg 3 times daily was initiated in new LNG 20 users when they had their first episode of bleeding or spotting, and treatment was continued until the day after the episode stopped. No significant reduction in median bleeding/spotting days when compared with placebo was seen.[20]

Antifibrinolytic agents

Tranexamic acid 500 mg 3 times daily was initiated in new LNG 20 IUD users when they had their first episode of bleeding or spotting, and treatment was continued until the day after the episode stopped. A reduction of 8 bleeding/spotting days over a 90-day period was noted ($P = .049$), but this was not significant after adjustment.[20]

Table 2					
Efficacy of medical interventions for irregular bleeding/spotting in LNG IUD users					
	Medication Class	**Medication**	**Dose (mg)**	**Frequency**	**Length of Time**
Decreased bleeding	NSAID	Naproxen	500	2 Times daily	5 d
	Antifibrinolytic	Tranexamic acid	500	3 Times daily	Until bleeding stops
	Antiprogestin	Mifepristone	100	Once	Monthly
No effect on bleeding	NSAID	Mefenamic acid	500	3 Times daily	Until bleeding stops
Increased bleeding	Estrogen	Estradiol	0.1	Transdermal	Changed weekly
	SPRM	Ulipristal acetate	50	Daily	3 d (Starting 21 d after insertion)

Estrogen

Estradiol has been studied as a means to stimulate endometrial estrogen receptors, with the goal of stabilizing the endometrial vasculature and epithelium. Clinical trials demonstrate estrogen is not an effective treatment of unscheduled bleeding. The estradiol 0.1-mg transdermal patch, beginning the day after LNG 20 IUD insertion and changed weekly for 12 weeks, was associated with an increase in bleeding and spotting days, with an adjusted relative risk of 1.25 (confidence interval 1.17–1.34). When the number of bleeding and spotting days were divided into quartiles, the estradiol group was most likely to be in the highest quartile when compared with placebo (40.9% vs 18.6%; $P = .02$). Four weeks after treatment, no difference in the number of bleeding or spotting days was noted. Dissatisfaction scores were higher in the estradiol group, with 39.5% reporting dissatisfaction with their bleeding pattern in the first 4 weeks compared with 11.6% of the placebo group.[19]

Antiprogestins

Antiprogestins like mifepristone inhibit progesterone, which leads to upregulation of endometrial estrogen receptors, inducing endometrial proliferation and theoretically reducing vaginal bleeding. Mifepristone 100 mg taken once on the day of insertion and repeated every 30 days for 3 cycles was associated with a significant decrease in median duration of intermenstrual bleeding or spotting episodes (6.0 vs 12.5 days; $P = .01$), as well as number of episodes (2.5 vs 3.0 episodes; $P = .05$). Three months after treatment, the median duration of intermenstrual bleeding remained lower in those who were treated with mifepristone (6 vs 15 days; $P = .008$). Satisfaction with the IUD was also higher in the treatment group, 75% versus 44% ($P = .004$).[21]

Mifepristone is most commonly used as part of a regimen for medical abortion and is available in 200-mg tablets. Mifepristone is not currently available as a lower dose, and the expense of this mediation makes it impractical now.

Selective progesterone receptor modulators

SPRMs like ulipristal acetate also bind with high affinity to the progesterone receptor, antagonizing the action of progesterone more selectively than mifepristone. Ulipristal acetate 50 mg daily for 3 days starting 3 weeks after IUD placement and repeated every 28 days was associated with a decrease in bleeding and spotting days after the first treatment (equivalent to 3 days less), but that effect was gone at the second cycle. By the third cycle, ulipristal treatment was associated with an increase in bleeding and spotting days, equivalent to 6 extra days.[22]

Summary of Recommendations for Unscheduled Bleeding with the Levonorgestrel Intrauterine Device

Reassurance should be the first-line recommendation for unscheduled bleeding in LNG IUD users. For those seeking medical intervention, modest evidence suggests decreased bleeding with naproxen and mifepristone, though low-dose mifepristone is not currently commercially available in the United States. One small trial with tranexamic acid suggests there may be some benefit. Other interventions are not recommended; mefenamic acid, transdermal estrogen, and ulipristal acetate either have no effect or increase bleeding.

ETONOGESTREL IMPLANT

The ENG implant (Implanon/Nexplanon [Merck & Co, Whitehouse Station, NJ, USA]) is associated with an overall decrease in bleeding, with 75% of women reporting fewer bleeding/spotting days after placement.[6] Over 3 months, 22% of ENG implant users will experience amenorrhea with the rest noting some form of unscheduled bleeding, including prolonged bleeding (17.7%) and frequent bleeding (6.7%).[6,23,24] Up to 23% of ENG implant users discontinue the device early because of bleeding concerns.[5] Another study revealed that 44% of women with unfavorable bleeding patterns (more bleeding/spotting days) over the first 3 months discontinued prematurely.[6] Risk factors for unscheduled bleeding have not been identified, though a favorable bleeding pattern in the first 3 months (few bleeding/spotting days) seems to predict a continued favorable pattern during the remainder of use. Even if an unfavorable bleeding pattern is present in the first 3 months, there is a 50% chance of improvement over time.[6]

Treatment of Irregular Bleeding

Studies addressing unscheduled bleeding with the ENG implant have focused on NSAIDs (ibuprofen and mefenamic acid), MMP inhibitors (doxycycline), antiprogestins (mifepristone), and estrogen. **Table 3** contains a summary of medical interventions shown to have a benefit in clinical trials for irregular bleeding in ENG implant users.

Limited data exist regarding treatment of unscheduled bleeding in ENG implant users, and most clinician recommendations are extrapolated from older data in Norplant (LNG implant) users. Based on data from Norplant, the US selected practice recommendations (SPR) for contraceptive use (2013) suggests NSAIDs for 5 to 7 days.[25] The US SPR for contraceptive use (2013) also recommends low-dose oral contraceptive pills or estrogen alone for 10 to 20 days if there are no contraindications to estrogen, though this approach has not been studied with the ENG implant. Use of cyclic combined oral contraceptives may help to promote scheduled bleeding during the placebo week and decrease unscheduled bleeding but may lead to more days of bleeding overall. Evidence from Norplant trials also suggests a benefit from cyclic oral progestins like medroxyprogesterone acetate 10 mg twice daily for 21 days followed by a 7-day pill-free interval for up to 3 months, progestin only pills, or tranexamic acid 500 mg twice daily for 5 days.[26,27]

Nonsteroidal antiinflammatory drugs

A retrospective cohort study used a chart review to see if the ENG implant removal rate differed for patients who presented for bleeding concerns and were offered reassurance alone or reassurance and an additional medical intervention. Thirty-three percent of those who had an implant placed returned to the office for bleeding concerns. Of those with bleeding concerns, 70% to 75% ultimately discontinued

Table 3					
Efficacy of medical interventions for irregular bleeding/spotting in ENG implant users					
	Medication Class	**Medication**	**Dose**	**Frequency**	**Length of Time**
Decreased bleeding	NSAID	Mefenamic acid	500 mg	3 Times daily	5 d
	MMPI	Doxycycline	100 mg	2 Times daily	5 d
	Antiprogestin combination	Mifepristone	25 mg	2 Times daily	1 d, then
		Estradiol	20 mcg	Daily	4 d
		Mifepristone	25 mg	2 Times daily	1 d, then
		Doxycycline	100 mg	2 Times daily	5 d
No effect on bleeding	Antiprogestin	Mifepristone	25 mg	2 Times daily	1 d
	MMPI and estradiol	Doxycycline	100 mg	2 Times daily	Both for 5 d
		Estradiol	20 mcg	Daily	

Abbreviation: MMPI, MMP inhibitors.

the implant early because of dissatisfaction with the bleeding pattern; the discontinuation rate did not differ whether the patients were offered reassurance alone or reassurance with ibuprofen.[28]

Mefenamic acid 500 mg 3 times daily for 5 days was given to ENG implant users who reported irregular bleeding and was associated with fewer bleeding or spotting episodes over the subsequent 4 weeks when compared with placebo (10.5 days vs 16.8 days; $P<.05$). Mefenamic acid users were also more likely to have the bleeding stop within 1 week (65.2% vs 21.7%; $P<.05$) and have a bleeding-free interval of more than 20 days over the next 28-day period (56.5% vs 21.7%; $P<.05$).[29]

Matrix metalloproteinase inhibitors

MMPs are expressed in the endometrium and play a role in endometrial tissue remodeling. MMP inhibitors like doxycycline inhibit the MMP-mediated matrix degradation and are thereby thought to help prevent unscheduled bleeding.

In a retrospective cohort study using a chart review to identify ENG implant removal rates when women with bleeding concerns were offered reassurance alone or an undisclosed doxycycline regimen, 75.5% discontinued their device early with reassurance alone, whereas those given reassurance and prescribed doxycycline had a significantly lower discontinuation rate for bleeding dissatisfaction (45.5%) ($P = .005$).[28]

Doxycycline 100 mg twice daily for 5 days was given to women with the ENG implant experiencing prolonged or frequent bleeding or spotting, with instructions to start treatment on day 2 of a bleeding episode. Time to bleeding cessation, including the first day of treatment, was 4.8 days for the doxycycline group compared with 7.5 days with placebo ($P = .001$). However, this benefit did not have an impact on subsequent bleeding patterns.[30] Another trial of doxycycline 100 mg twice daily for 5 days was given in the same patient population but was not associated with a decrease in time to bleeding cessation (6.4 days for both doxycycline and placebo), though that trial was inadequately powered (204 participants, 490 required for 80% power and alpha of 0.05).[31]

Antiprogestins

Mifepristone 25 mg twice daily for 1 day was given to women with the ENG implant who had prolonged or frequent bleeding, initiated on the second day of a bleeding episode. Mifepristone was not significantly associated with a change in time to bleeding cessation (5.9 days mifepristone, 7.5 days placebo; $P = .283$).[30] As mentioned previously, mifepristone is not commercially available in a 25-mg dose, and providing the currently available 200-mg dose makes this intervention cost prohibitive.

Combination therapy: antiprogestins, estrogen, and matrix metalloproteinase inhibitors

Mifepristone 25 mg twice daily for 1 day followed by estradiol 20 mcg daily for 4 days was given to women with the ENG implant experiencing prolonged or frequent bleeding starting on the second day of a bleeding episode. Although mifepristone alone did not decrease time to bleeding cessation in this study by Weisberg and colleagues,[30] mifepristone with estradiol was associated with a significant decrease in time to bleeding cessation (4.2 days vs 7.5 days in the placebo group; $P<.001$). Despite a benefit in the current bleeding episode, subsequent bleeding episodes were not delayed or shortened. In a second, larger study with 5 study groups, Weisberg and colleagues[31] noted similar results. Women randomized to receive mifepristone 25 mg twice daily for 1 day followed by estradiol 20 mcg daily for 4 days had a significant decrease in time to bleeding cessation (4 days vs 6.4 days placebo; $P = .0008$).

Mifepristone 25 mg twice daily for 1 day followed by doxycycline 100 mg twice daily for 5 days was given to another study group on the second day of a bleeding episode. This group also had a significant decrease in time to bleeding cessation (4.4 days vs 6.4 days placebo; $P = .01$). Doxycycline 100 mg twice daily with estradiol 20 mcg daily for 5 days was not associated with a change in time to bleeding cessation (6.4 days for both treatment and placebo groups).[31]

None of the combination therapies had an effect on subsequent bleeding patterns beyond the treatment period.[31]

Summary of Recommendations for Unscheduled Bleeding with the Etonogestrel Implant

Reassurance should be the first line in the treatment of irregular bleeding in ENG implant users. For those seeking medical intervention, modest evidence suggests use of mefenamic acid, mifepristone with estradiol, mifepristone with doxycycline, or doxycycline alone. Mifepristone alone was not associated with a decrease in bleeding. Despite being associated with a decrease in bleeding when used alone, doxycycline in combination with estradiol was not associated with a significant change.

SUMMARY

LARC devices, such as IUDs and implants, are the most effective reversible contraceptives available and have few contraindications. Changes in bleeding patterns after placement are a leading cause of early discontinuation. **Fig. 1** is an algorithm on how to address dissatisfaction with bleeding profiles after device placement. Use of NSAIDs can be recommended to decrease bleeding with all LARC devices and tranexamic acid for either IUD. In addition to these recommendations, consider

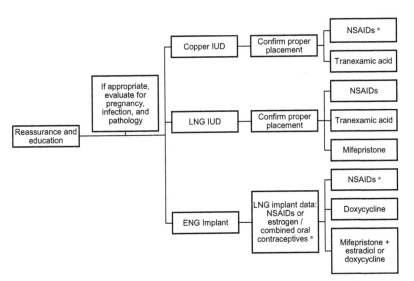

Fig. 1. Management algorithm of bleeding concerns in LARC users. [a]Endorsed by the US SPR for contraceptive use (2013).

additional estrogen, combined oral contraceptives, or progesterone as extrapolated from Norplant (LNG implant) studies and clinician experience, though no data currently support or refute its use with currently available LARC devices. More research needs to be done in this area to try to improve bleeding patterns and user satisfaction with these highly effective methods.

REFERENCES

1. American College of Obstetricians and Gynecologists. ACOG practice bulletin No. 121: long-acting reversible contraception: implants and intrauterine devices. Obstet Gynecol 2011;118:184–96.
2. Moreau C, Cleland K, Trussell J. Contraceptive discontinuation attributed to method dissatisfaction in the United States. Contraception 2007;76:267–72.
3. Bayer Healthcare Pharmaceuticals Inc. Skyla prescribing information. 2013. Available at: http://labeling.bayerhealthcare.com/html/products/pi/Skyla_PI.pdf. Accessed August 17, 2015.
4. Sivin I, Stern J. Health during prolonged use of levonorgestrel 20 micrograms/d and the copper TCu 380Ag intrauterine contraceptive devices: a multicenter study. International Committee for Contraception Research (ICCR). Fertil Steril 1994;61:70–7.
5. Casey PM, Long ME, Marnach ML, et al. Bleeding related to etonogestrel subdermal implant in a US population. Contraception 2011;83:426–30.
6. Mansour D, Korver T, Marintcheva-Petrova M, et al. The effects of Implanon on menstrual bleeding patterns. Eur J Contracept Reprod Health Care 2008; 13(Suppl 1):13–28.
7. Makarainen L, Ylikorkala O. Ibuprofen prevents IUCD-induced increases in menstrual blood loss. Br J Obstet Gynaecol 1986;93:285–8.
8. Suvisaari J, Lahteenmaki P. Detailed analysis of menstrual bleeding patterns after postmenstrual and postabortal insertion of a copper IUD or a levonorgestrel-releasing intrauterine system. Contraception 1996;54:201–8.
9. Champion CB, Behlilovic B, Arosemena JM, et al. A three-year evaluation of TCu 380 Ag and multiload Cu 375 intrauterine devices. Contraception 1988;38: 631–9.
10. Roy S, Shaw ST Jr. Role of prostaglandins in IUD-associated uterine bleeding–effect of a prostaglandin synthetase inhibitor (ibuprofen). Obstet Gynecol 1981;58:101–6.
11. Toppozada M. Treatment of increased menstrual blood loss in IUD users. Contraception 1987;36:145–57.
12. Wu S, Wang C, Cheng W, et al. Randomized multi-center study of baofuxin for treatment of bleeding side-effect induced by IUD. Reprod Contracept 2000;11: 152–7.
13. Pizarro E, Mehech G, Hidalgo M, et al. Effect of meclofenamic acid on menstruation in hypermenorrheic women using intrauterine devices. Rev Chil Obstet Ginecol 1988;53:43–56 [in Spanish].
14. Mercorio F, De Simone R, Di Carlo C, et al. Effectiveness and mechanism of action of desmopressin in the treatment of copper intrauterine device-related menorrhagia: a pilot study. Hum Reprod 2003;18:2319–22.
15. Ylikorkala O, Viinikka L. Comparison between antifibrinolytic and antiprostaglandin treatment in the reduction of increased menstrual blood loss in women with intrauterine contraceptive devices. Br J Obstet Gynaecol 1983;90:78–83.
16. Pedron N, Lozano M, Gallegos AJ. The effect of acetylsalicylic acid on menstrual blood loss in women with IUDs. Contraception 1987;36:295–303.

17. Lin X, Gao ES, Li D, et al. Preventive treatment of intrauterine device-induced menstrual blood loss with tranexamic acid in Chinese women. Acta Obstet Gynecol Scand 2007;86:1126–9.
18. Hidalgo M, Bahamondes L, Perrotti M, et al. Bleeding patterns and clinical performance of the levonorgestrel-releasing intrauterine system (Mirena) up to two years. Contraception 2002;65:129–32.
19. Madden T, Proehl S, Allsworth JE, et al. Naproxen or estradiol for bleeding and spotting with the levonorgestrel intrauterine system: a randomized controlled trial. Am J Obstet Gynecol 2012;206(129):e1–8.
20. Sordal T, Inki P, Draeby J, et al. Management of initial bleeding or spotting after levonorgestrel-releasing intrauterine system placement: a randomized controlled trial. Obstet Gynecol 2013;121:934–41.
21. Lal S, Kriplani A, Kulshrestha V, et al. Efficacy of mifepristone in reducing intermenstrual vaginal bleeding in users of the levonorgestrel intrauterine system. Int J Gynaecol Obstet 2010;109:128–30.
22. Warner P, Guttinger A, Glasier AF, et al. Randomized placebo-controlled trial of CDB-2914 in new users of a levonorgestrel-releasing intrauterine system shows only short-lived amelioration of unscheduled bleeding. Hum Reprod 2010;25:345–53.
23. Darney P, Patel A, Rosen K, et al. Safety and efficacy of a single-rod etonogestrel implant (Implanon): results from 11 international clinical trials. Fertil Steril 2009;91:1646–53.
24. Zheng SR, Zheng HM, Qian SZ, et al. A randomized multicenter study comparing the efficacy and bleeding pattern of a single-rod (Implanon) and a six-capsule (Norplant) hormonal contraceptive implant. Contraception 1999;60:1–8.
25. Division of Reproductive Health, National Center for Chronic Disease Prevention and Health Promotion, Centers for Disease Control and Prevention (CDC). U.S. selected practice recommendations for contraceptive use, 2013: adapted from the World Health Organization selected practice recommendations for contraceptive use, 2nd edition. MMWR Recomm Rep 2013;62:1–60.
26. Mansour D, Bahamondes L, Critchley H, et al. The management of unacceptable bleeding patterns in etonogestrel-releasing contraceptive implant users. Contraception 2011;83:202–10.
27. Phupong V, Sophonsritsuk A, Taneepanichskul S. The effect of tranexamic acid for treatment of irregular uterine bleeding secondary to Norplant use. Contraception 2006;73:253–6.
28. Casey PM, Long ME, Drozdowicz LB, et al. Management of etonogestrel subdermal implant-related bleeding. J Reprod Med 2014;59:306–12.
29. Phaliwong P, Taneepanichskul S. The effect of mefenamic acid on controlling irregular uterine bleeding second to Implanon use. J Med Assoc Thai 2004;87(Suppl 3):S64–8.
30. Weisberg E, Hickey M, Palmer D, et al. A pilot study to assess the effect of three short-term treatments on frequent and/or prolonged bleeding compared to placebo in women using Implanon. Hum Reprod 2006;21:295–302.
31. Weisberg E, Hickey M, Palmer D, et al. A randomized controlled trial of treatment options for troublesome uterine bleeding in Implanon users. Hum Reprod 2009;24:1852–61.

Contraceptive Coverage and the Affordable Care Act

Mary Tschann, MPH*, Reni Soon, MD, MPH

KEYWORDS

- Affordable Care Act • Contraception • Mandate • Medicaid • Contraceptive access
- Legal challenges

KEY POINTS

- The Patient Protection and Affordable Care Act (ACA) was signed into law by President Obama on March 23, 2010, with the primary goals of expanding access to insurance coverage and reducing health care spending.
- A major underpinning of the legislation was shifting the focus of both health care and insurance providers away from reactive medical care toward preventive care, and to meet this goal, the ACA required health insurers to provide preventive health care, including the full range of contraceptives, to patients without cost sharing.
- This article describes both the current landscape of contraceptive coverage in the United States after the implementation of the contraceptive mandate and the delays and inconsistencies related to its implementation to date.

INTRODUCTION

The Affordable Care Act, Preventative Health Care, and Contraception

The ACA was signed into law by President Obama on March 23, 2010, with the primary goals of expanding access to insurance coverage and reducing health care spending. A major underpinning of the legislation was shifting the focus of both health care and insurance providers away from reactive medical care toward preventive care.

Public health advocates have long recognized that the most successful health care systems are those that focus on primary prevention of disease, rather than on treatment of acute illnesses. Specifically, an analysis in the United States of preventive health care services, such as tobacco cessation screening and immunizations, showed that these programs saved 2 million life-years at minimal cost.[1] Such studies serve as the foundation for the ACA's goal of pivoting the US health

Department of Obstetrics, Gynecology, and Women's Health, University of Hawaii John A. Burns School of Medicine, 1319 Punahou Street, Suite 824, Honolulu, HI 96826, USA
* Corresponding author.
E-mail address: mtschann@hawaii.edu

Obstet Gynecol Clin N Am 42 (2015) 605–617
http://dx.doi.org/10.1016/j.ogc.2015.07.001
0889-8545/15/$ – see front matter © 2015 Elsevier Inc. All rights reserved.
obgyn.theclinics.com

care system toward prevention of disease and promotion of overall health and well-being.

To actualize this goal, the ACA stipulated that insurers may not apply cost sharing (co-pays, co-insurance, or deductibles) to a panel of preventive services. These services include high blood pressure and cholesterol screening, testing for sexually transmitted infections, alcohol misuse and abuse screening and counseling, and a variety of cancer screenings and immunizations. The ACA preventive services coverage mandate also included specific preventive care for women.

When the ACA was signed in 2010, the value of covering preventive health care services was well recognized. Many private sector insurance payors were already covering preventive services: all 50 states required plans to cover mammography screening, and 29 states required plans to cover cervical cancer screening.[2]

After the signing of the ACA, the Department of Health and Human Services (HHS) tasked the Institute of Medicine (IOM) with determining which services should be included as preventive health care services under the ACA. The IOM convened the Committee on Preventive Services for Women, which comprised experts from diverse fields in medicine, public health, and health policy. In 2011, this committee released its recommendations on which services should be covered by the ACA.[2] This list included "the full range of Food and Drug Administration (FDA)-approved contraceptive methods, sterilization procedures, and patient education and counseling for women with reproductive capacity." The HHS adopted these recommendations, and implementation of this provision began in August 2012.

Although some question the need for including contraception as a component of general preventive services for women, the public health benefits of preventing unintended pregnancy are pronounced and well established. Every year in the United States, 600 to 700 women die because of complications associated with pregnancy,[3] and the maternal mortality ratio (MMR) in the United States continues to increase.[3] In a recent examination of US pregnancy-related mortality, the MMR was 16.0 per 100,000 live births for the period 2006–2010.[3] Another analysis of global maternal mortality found that the US MMR in 2013 was 18.5 per 100,000 live births, which is comparable to the ratio in countries with fewer health care resources, including Turkey, Russia, Iran, and Romania.[4] Reducing unintended pregnancy is an important element of addressing the unacceptably high MMR in the United States.

In addition, there are well-established negative health and socioeconomic outcomes associated with unplanned births. Unplanned pregnancies are associated with delayed initiation of prenatal care and a decreased likelihood of breast-feeding.[5] Short spacing between pregnancies increases the risk of negative birth outcomes, namely, preterm birth and low-birth-weight babies.[6,7] Moreover, the ability to plan pregnancies allows women the time and finances to invest in their own education and careers and participate more fully in the workforce, benefitting not only themselves and their families but also the society as a whole.[8,9]

Unintended pregnancies may risk the health and well-being of women and their families, and the financial implications of unintended pregnancy are also substantial. Including only the medical costs of an unplanned pregnancy and 1 year of life of the child, the Brookings Institute, a nonpartisan public policy group, estimated that the cost to taxpayers of publicly funded unintended pregnancies and the infants born of those pregnancies averaged $11 billion annually.[10]

Although the contraceptive coverage mandate has proved to be a highly divisive issue, it is not a provision unique to the ACA. By the time the ACA was signed, government-funded insurance had already been covering contraception for decades. More than half of states had laws requiring that insurance plans cover contraceptive methods even before ACA implementation.[11] In 2002, the most recent year before the ACA with data available, more than 89% of insurance plans covered contraception,[11] and in a 2010 survey of employers, FDA-approved contraceptives were reported to be covered by 85% of large employers and 62% of small employers.[12]

Medicaid Expansion and Family Planning

Another component of the ACA was the loosening of eligibility requirements for Medicaid family planning services. For approximately the last 20 years, states have had the option of increasing the income threshold or establishing other criteria by which individuals could access low- or no-cost family planning services through the Medicaid waiver program. The waiver program was a mechanism for creating demonstration projects that both expand services and provide a real-world analysis of a project's feasibility and impact on beneficiaries. States receive funding to support the projects, but funding is contingent on periodic reapplication and approval by the Centers for Medicaid and Medicare Services.[13] These projects have been immensely effective at reducing unintended pregnancies,[14] increasing uptake of highly effective contraceptive methods,[15] and improving pregnancy spacing,[16] while also being highly cost-effective.[17] These programs have been shown to produce cost savings of up to $159 million annually.[18]

As the ACA was being developed, the success of expanded family planning waiver programs was apparent, and many of these had moved beyond being demonstration projects to become integral parts of a state's family planning services. In light of this success, legislators created a mechanism in the ACA by which these programs could be permanently integrated into state's Medicaid plans. States that choose to make their expanded access to family planning permanent may now do so through a State Plan Amendment (SPA). SPAs are implemented state by state, and therefore their eligibility requirements vary, but all are tied to consumer income, with eligibility ranging from approximately 140% to 300% of Federal Poverty Level (FPL).[19]

The ACA provided funds for the expansion of Medicaid in general to all individuals making up to 138% of the FPL. Before the ACA, each state dictated coverage eligibility for its own Medicaid program. However, as discussed later, the Supreme Court determined that the federal government could not require states to expand their Medicaid programs, which effectively made this intended expansion optional for states. If all states participated in the expansion, an additional 17 million low-income individuals who otherwise would not have qualified for Medicaid would have coverage.[20] Because Medicaid provides for full coverage of family planning services, increasing access to Medicaid also expands access to contraception.

Contraceptive Coverage Mandate Goal: Reducing Barriers to Effective Prevention

Although coverage of contraception was already standard practice in most private health insurance plans and government-funded insurance, the ACA was groundbreaking in that it stipulated that this coverage could not include any co-payments, deductibles, or other cost sharing by patients; this is significant in light of recent evidence showing that co-payments are a barrier to accessing contraception, particularly the most effective methods of contraception, which typically have substantial up-front costs.[21]

Several studies have shown that with counseling and removal of logistical and financial obstacles, such as prohibitive cost sharing, most women will choose the most effective methods of contraception.[22,23] In a prospective study in St Louis, more than 9000 women were provided with contraceptive counseling and the method of their choice at no cost.[23,24] About 75% of the women chose an intrauterine device

(IUD) or an implant, which is markedly higher than the national IUD and implant use rate of 7.2%,[25] and subsequent analyses have shown a decrease in the unintended pregnancies, abortions, and teen births in this population.[24,26]

Trussel and colleagues[27] created an economic model to estimate the potential savings if more women in the United States. switched to highly effective methods of contraception, such as IUDs and implants. They found that if just 10% of women aged 20 to 29 years switched from oral contraception to an implant or IUD, the cost savings would be approximately $288 million each year.

The current landscape of contraceptive coverage in the United States after the enactment of the contraceptive mandate and the delays and inconsistencies related to its implementation to date are described in the following.

STATUS OF THE CONTRACEPTIVE COVERAGE MANDATE IMPLEMENTATION: PROGRESS AND DELAYS
No-Cost Contraceptive Coverage Expansion

As the contraceptive coverage mandate went into effect in August 2012, there is as yet no extensive evidence regarding its impact. However, recent Guttmacher analysis found that since the implementation of the contraceptive coverage mandate, out-of-pocket costs for contraception for privately insured women have been substantially reduced. The proportion of privately insured women paying out of pocket for oral contraception decreased from 85% in the fall of 2012 to 33% in spring of 2014.[28] Among women who reported using IUDs, the proportion who paid nothing for their method increased from 45% in the fall of 2012 to 62% in the spring of 2014. The estimated cost savings in 2013 related to the contraceptive mandate was more than $483 million in out-of-pocket costs, an average of $269 per woman.[29]

Medicaid Expansion and Expanded Contraceptive Access

As of July 2015, 29 states and the District of Columbia have adopted Medicaid expansion under the ACA.[30] Since the beginning of 2014, 8 million additional women have obtained insurance through expanded Medicaid coverage.[31] Because the ACA was written with the expectation that all states would have expanded coverage through Medicaid, in states that have declined to expand coverage there exists a large gap in coverage options for individuals whose income is more than the threshold for their state's Medicaid but less than the minimum required to qualify for federal health insurance premiums. In states that have not chosen to expand their Medicaid coverage, 4 million people are in the coverage gap, and 49% of these individuals are women.[32]

A total of 29 states have expanded access to family planning through Medicaid waiver or SPAs. The authors found no published analysis of the increased enrollment or corresponding increase in contraceptive uptake associated with these programs since the signing of the ACA, but an analysis in 2011 predicted that the states without an SPA could serve up to 100,000 women each and save between $2.3 million and $17.4 million dollars per year if they were to establish a program.[33]

Limitations and Inconsistencies with Mandate Compliance

Grandfathered plans
To promote a smooth implementation, the ACA provided for tiered adoption of certain components of the legislation by some insurance plans. This accommodation, known as grandfathering, allows plans that were already in existence at the time the ACA was signed into law to continue to apply cost sharing to preventive services. Plans maintain their grandfathered status as long as they impose no increases in patient cost sharing through premiums, deductibles, or co-pays.[34] These plans are

quickly disappearing; employees covered by a grandfathered plan dropped from 48% in 2012 to 26% in 2014.[35] Employers are also reducing the number of grandfathered plans offered to employees, with 54% offering at least 1 grandfathered plan to employees in 2013, down from 72% in 2011.[35]

Inconsistencies in compliance

Inconsistencies in interpretation and compliance with the contraceptive mandate have been confirmed by recent research. A report by Sonfield[36] found that some plans are not providing full coverage for the entire range of contraceptive methods available, particularly for coverage of IUD and injectable contraceptives. This same study found that some plans are declining to provide coverage for the contraceptive patch and ring because they have the same hormonal ingredients used in oral contraceptives,[36] even though the FDA classifies these as distinct methods because of their different modes of delivery.[37] Similarly, a recent review of coverage for emergency contraception (EC) among the largest insurers in the state of Hawaii revealed that the predominance of plans were still applying cost sharing for the 3 types of FDA-approved EC—levonorgestrel, ulipristal acetate, and the copper IUD (de Silva KL, unpublished data, 2015).

A Kaiser Foundation report reinforced these findings. Through an analysis of 20 insurance carriers in 5 states, California, Georgia, Michigan, New Jersey, and Texas, significant variability was seen for coverage of 12 prescribed contraceptive methods. Only 12 of the 20 insurers reported covering the contraceptive ring with no cost sharing, whereas only 10 of the 20 insurers cover all FDA-approved IUDs without limitations or cost sharing, and 1 carrier in the study does not cover the Paragard IUD, the only nonhormonal IUD, at all.[38]

In response to these inconsistencies, HHS published new guidance for insurers and consumers in May 2015.[39] These guidelines, outlined in **Table 1**, specifically delineate the methods of contraception that must be covered without cost sharing. The guidelines confirm that plans must offer at least 1 method with no cost sharing within each of the categories (currently 18) of contraception identified by the FDA and that coverage cannot be restricted based on the plan offering other methods that are "medically appropriate" for a patient.

Under the new guidance, plans are still allowed to use "reasonable medical management techniques" to regulate costs. Commonly used management techniques include tiered drug formularies that allow cost sharing for brand-name pharmaceuticals when a generic is available or the collection of co-pays and deductibles if services are received outside of the preferred provider network.[39] However, the new guidelines clarify the boundaries of these techniques and reinforce that plans must also have an "easily accessible, transparent, and sufficiently expedient exceptions process" for methods deemed to be medically necessary by the provider. There is no generic equivalent for many contraceptive methods approved by the FDA, including the contraceptive ring, ulipristal acetate EC, implant, and IUDs, so this specific medical management technique should not be applied to these methods.

Legal Challenges to the Affordable Care Act

In both its development and implementation, the ACA has been steeped in debate and disagreement. Although Congress has made efforts to repeal or eliminate certain provisions of the law, the political tug-of-war regarding the ACA has been primarily focused in the courts. Within minutes of the law being signed by President Obama, the first lawsuit challenging the law's constitutionality was filed.[40]

At present, 150 cases have been filed regarding the ACA.[41] These cases may be grouped into 2 broad categories: cases aimed to repeal the ACA in its entirety and

Method	Coverage Required	FDA-Approved Methods[a]
Contraceptive implant	X	Nexplanon/Implanon
Progestin IUD	X	Mirena/Skyla/Liletta
Copper IUD	X	Paragard
Injectable contraception	X	Generics available
Progestin-only oral contraceptive	X	Generics available
Combined hormonal oral contraceptive	X	Generics available
Extended use oral contraceptive	X	Generics available
Contraceptive patch	X	Xulane[b] generic available
Contraceptive ring	X	NuvaRing
Emergency contraception (levonorgestrel)	X	NextChoice generic available
Emergency contraception (ulipristal acetate)	X	Ella
Diaphragm	X	Milex Omniflex
Cervical cap	X	FemCap
Contraceptive sponge	X	Today sponge[c]
Female condom	X	Multiple types[c]
Spermicide	X	Multiple types[c]
Sterilization, tubal ligation	X	N/A
Sterilization, implant	X	Essure

Table 1
Contraceptive methods for women currently identified by the FDA

[a] Plans must cover at least 1 method in each category; may be generic.
[b] OthroEvra being discontinued by manufacturer; Xulane generic introduced in April 2014.
[c] Over-the-counter products covered with valid prescription.
Data from Departments of Labor (DOL), Health and Human Services (HHS), and the Treasury. FAQS about Affordable Care Act implementation (part XXVI), May 11, 2015. Available at: http://www.cms.gov/CCIIO/Resources/Fact-Sheets-and-FAQs/Downloads/aca_implementation_faqs26.pdf. Accessed July 16, 2015.

cases focused specifically on eliminating or refining the contraceptive coverage mandate. The authors briefly review seminal cases regarding the ACA as a whole and then focus on legal challenges aimed specifically at the contraceptive coverage mandate.

Overall Challenges to Affordable Care Act Implementation

In National Federation of Independent Businesses v Sebelius, decided in 2012, the Supreme Court upheld the constitutionality of the individual insurance coverage mandate component of the ACA, thereby validating the central tenet of the legislation. In the same decision, however, the Supreme Court limited the scope of the ACA substantially by ruling that the Medicaid expansion provisions of the ACA, which required that states expand Medicaid to cover nonelderly, nondisabled adults with income less than 138% of the FPL, were coercive.[42] This case confirmed the fundamental constitutionality of the ACA, and it also allowed states to choose whether or not to participate in the Medicaid expansion. As of July 2015, nineteen states have refused the expansion.

A second series of cases (consolidated as King v Burwell) was decided by the Supreme Court in June 2015.[43] The plaintiffs in this case were disputing the federal government's right to grant health insurance premium subsidies to individuals who have purchased their health insurance from the federal, rather than a state-run, health insurance exchange. This challenge is derived from a single line of text in the law that describes those eligible for the subsidies as individuals who purchase their insurance through state-run exchanges. The Court decided against the plaintiffs, determining that when read in context, the statutory language was clearly intended to treat the federal and state-run exchanges equally under the law, meaning that taxpayers who purchase their insurance through either type of exchange are eligible for subsidies. Had the Court sided with the plaintiffs, consumers in 36 states would have lost their access to health insurance subsidies, which the Court determined would destabilize the individual insurance market in those states and cause the very kind of market volatility that the ACA was designed to prevent.

Contraceptive Coverage Mandate Legal Challenges

By far the largest proportion of legal challenges to the ACA has focused on the contraceptive coverage mandate embedded in the preventive services provision. To date, 101 cases have been filed challenging the mandate.[41] These challenges cite both an infringement of the religious freedom guarantees of the First Amendment and of the Religious Freedom Restoration Act of 1993 (RFRA). RFRA states that the "government shall not substantially burden a person's exercise of religion." The corporations and organizations filing suit claim that the requirement to provide contraceptive coverage in their health plans is a violation of their rights under RFRA.

HHS has responded to these concerns through clarifications and changes to the law (**Table 2** for a list of these accommodations). As of 2012, religious institutions that are primarily houses of worship are fully exempted from the requirement to provide contraceptive coverage in their insurance plans. To qualify for exemption, an organization must meet specific criteria under the federal tax code. The predominance of institutions that meet these criteria is churches, synagogues, or other houses of worship.[44]

These narrow inclusion criteria were purposeful.[45] It is intended to limit the exemption for this requirement only to those organizations whose primary goal is the inculcation of specific religious values and who are most likely to employ individuals who share the same religious values as the organization; this is in contrast to other religiously affiliated organizations, such as hospitals and universities, that often employ or educate large numbers of individuals of a variety of religious backgrounds. HHS argues that employees and students in these organizations should not have their access to the full breadth of preventive health services guaranteed by the ACA limited because of the views of their employer or institution.

After concerns were expressed by these religiously affiliated organizations, HHS issued revised rules that provided for an accommodation, but not an exemption, for these plans.[46] This accommodation allowed these institutions to notify their insurance carrier of their objection to providing contraception, at which point the insurance carrier assumes responsibility for providing this coverage to the individual directly. The nonprofit itself therefore is not required to pay for, facilitate, or participate in any of the transactions associated with the employee obtaining contraception. Despite these accommodations, challenges to the mandate continue.

Challenges brought by nonprofit organizations

At present, 46 nonprofit institutions have filed suit over the contraceptive mandate.[41] Some religiously affiliated institutions have argued that the act of completing the self-certification form violates their moral values as it facilitates employees obtaining contraception. Circuit courts have disagreed about the merits of this claim (Michigan v Burwell and Roman Catholic Archbishop v Sebelius), but in an unsigned decision in

Table 2
Current exemptions and accommodations for the Affordable Care Act

Category	Applies To	Description	Effective Since
Grandfathered plans	Plans that insured at least 1 person as of March 23, 2010, and have not made any changes to benefits since that time (including any increases in cost/cost sharing)	Plans do not have to adhere to no-cost sharing preventive services regulations	2010
Full exemption from coverage	Houses of worship (eg, churches, synagogues)	Fully exempt from providing coverage for contraceptives	2012
Accommodation: nonprofit	Nonprofit institutions that have a religious objection to providing some or all contraceptives	Institutions can self-certify (via completion of a form sent to insurer or a letter sent to HHS) their religious objection. Coverage for contraception managed and paid for entirely by insurer	2013: Self-certification form 2014: Option to submit letter directly to HHS
Accommodation: closely held corporations	Closely held corporations	Closely held corporations can use the same accommodations that are available to nonprofit organizations	Pending: provisional rules introduced in 2014; awaiting final rules with definition for closely held and instructions for self-certifying

2014, the Supreme Court supported Wheaton College's argument that completing the form was a violation of its religious values[47] and granted an injunction. In its decision, the Supreme Court agreed with the institution that it should not have to complete a form to certify that it has moral objections to providing contraception, and instead the institution could simply inform the HHS in writing that they qualified for an exemption. HHS would then bear the responsibility for arranging third party coverage for these methods via the institution's insurance carrier. In a strongly worded rebuttal, dissenting justices noted that this decision will create additional confusion and new layers of bureaucracy in an already complicated system. HHS recently released new guidelines for nonprofits (see **Table 2**) in response to this ruling.

Challenges brought by for-profit institutions

A slightly larger number of challenges (49 at present[42]) to the contraceptive coverage mandate are from for-profit organizations. For-profit organizations were not included in the religious accommodations in the ACA as, historically, corporations were not considered capable of practicing religion. In these suits, for-profit employers have argued that covering some or all contraceptive methods violates their religious beliefs and contend that they should not be required to provide their employees with health care plans that offer such coverage.

In June 2014, the Supreme Court issued their decision in the primary case for this issue, Burwell v Hobby Lobby. In a 5-to-4 decision, the Court decided that closely held corporations, defined as those with a limited number of shareholders, can assert protections under RFRA. The Court majority stated that the owners' belief that their religious freedom was being burdened was sufficient cause to warrant an accommodation by the government. Because HHS had created accommodations for nonprofit organizations, the Court reasoned that the same accommodations could be extended to closely held corporations that expressed a religious objection to providing contraceptive coverage.

However, as mentioned previously, the Supreme Court issued an injunction on the implementation of this accommodation for Wheaton College a few days after the Hobby Lobby decision. At present, the administration is accepting public comment on and finalizing new rules in response to these regulations that would allow closely held for-profit companies to register their objection to the contraceptive coverage mandate. At question are definitions of closely held corporations and the mechanism by which for-profit organizations should be required to certify their objection to the contraceptive mandate.[44] In the meantime, women in these insurance plans are in limbo when it comes to coverage for some contraceptive methods.

Table 2 shows the current list of coverage exemptions and accommodations for employer-sponsored health insurance. This list will continue to evolve as new rules are introduced.

Discussion

Pending legal challenges to the ACA and the contraceptive mandate indicate that additional developments in contraceptive coverage are likely. Despite this, already there are benefits from the mandate in the number of privately insured women who are obtaining their methods without cost sharing. As discussed earlier, eliminating cost as a barrier to highly effective methods of contraception is associated with increased uptake of those methods, which in turn has been shown to contribute to reductions in unintended pregnancy and abortion rates.[23]

Despite the ongoing legal wrangling about the appropriateness of including contraception as a preventative health benefit, evidence shows that coverage for contraception is popular among consumers. A recent study found that 69% of respondents to a nationally representative survey expressed support for requiring employers to provide insurance coverage for contraception.[48] Another study of religiously affiliated women found universally high levels of support for requiring insurers to cover contraception.[49]

A most troubling result of the evolving nature of the contraceptive coverage mandate is the increased difficulty faced by patients and their providers in accessing insurance benefits. A large-scale national study demonstrated the challenges researchers faced in obtaining accurate information from insurance companies about contraceptive benefits.[38] Patients, particularly those who are young or nonnative English speakers, are likely to face even greater hurdles in trying to understand what their benefits are and whether they are being unfairly denied access to a method.

The challenges faced by patients are substantial enough that the National Women's Law Center (NWLC) has established a resource center to assist patients in navigating, understanding, and advocating for coverage of their birth control method. The NWLC has a Web site dedicated to assisting patients with this process (coverher.org) and has created a step-by-step guide for patients. NWLC reported that women from every state have contacted the center to obtain assistance in navigating a health care plan that was inappropriately denying coverage. The new guidance issued by HHS is a sign that plans may soon be using a standardized and more transparent process in interpreting the requirements and providing benefits.

Although it is difficult to yet tell the full impact of the ACA on contraceptive access, unintended pregnancy, unintended birth, and abortion, one has only to look at the benefits seen in public family planning programs to see the potential for substantial public health improvements in these areas. Publicly funded family planning has proved to be a huge cost-saving mechanism for states and a major resource in averting unintended pregnancy and abortion.[33] Lowering the persistently high unintended pregnancy rate will be transformative for women, families, and our communities. Expanded access to highly effective contraception through both public and private insurance is crucial to this effort.

REFERENCES

1. Maciosek MV, Coffield AB, Flottemesch TJ, et al. Greater use of preventive services in US health care could save lives at little or no cost. Health Aff 2010;29: 1656–60.
2. Institute of Medicine. Clinical preventive services for women: closing the gaps. Washington, DC: National Academies Press; 2011.
3. Creanga AA, Berg CJ, Syverson C, et al. Pregnancy-related mortality in the United States, 2006-2010. Obstet Gynecol 2015;125:5–12.
4. Kassebaum NJ, Bertozzi-Villa A, Coggeshall MS, et al. Global, regional, and national levels and causes of maternal mortality during 1990–2013: a systematic analysis for the Global Burden of Disease Study 2013. Lancet 2014;384: 980–1004.
5. Gipson JD, Koenig MA, Hindin MJ. The effects of unintended pregnancy on infant, child, and parental health: a review of the literature. Stud Fam Plann 2008; 39:18–38.
6. Conde-Agudelo A, Rosas-Bermúdez A, Kafury-Goeta AC. Birth spacing and risk of adverse perinatal outcomes: a meta-analysis. JAMA 2006;295:1809–23.
7. Zhu B-P. Effect of interpregnancy interval on birth outcomes: findings from three recent US studies. Int J Gynecol Obstet 2005;89:S25–33.

8. Goldin C, Katz LF. The power of the pill: oral contraceptives and women's career and marriage decisions. Cambridge (MA): National bureau of economic research; 2000.
9. Goldin C, Katz LF. Career and marriage in the age of the pill. Am Econ Rev 2000; 90:461–5.
10. Monea E, Thomas A. Unintended pregnancy and taxpayer spending. Perspect Sex Reprod Health 2011;43:88–93.
11. Sonfield A, Gold RB, Frost JJ, et al. US insurance coverage of contraceptives and the impact of contraceptive coverage mandates, 2002. Perspect Sex Reprod Health 2004;36:72–9.
12. Claxton G, DiJulio B, Finder B, et al. Employer health benefits. 2010 Annual Survey. Chicago (IL): Henry J. Kaiser Family Foundation; 2008.
13. Ranji U. Medicaid and family planning: background and implications of the ACA. Issue Brief. Chicago (IL): Henry J. Kaiser Family Foundation; 2015.
14. Biggs M, Foster D, Hulett D, et al. Cost-benefit analysis of the California Family PACT Program for calendar year 2007. San Francisco (CA): Bixby Center for Global Reproductive Health; 2010.
15. Cawthon L. Take charge final evaluation: first five years, July 2001-June 2006. Olympia (WA): Research and Data Analysis Division, Department of Social and Health Services; 2006.
16. Texas Health and Human Services Commission. Women's Health Program Annual Report. 2008. Available at: http://www.hhsc.state.tx.us/reports/2010/WHP_2008 AnnualReport.pdf. Accessed May 5, 2015.
17. Centers for Medicare and Medicaid Services. Family planning services option and new benefit rules for benchmark plans. State Medicaid Director Letter. Washington, DC: Department of Health and Human Services; 2010.
18. Edwards J, Bronstein J, Adams K. Evaluation of Medicaid family planning demonstrations. CMS Contract No. 752-2-415921. Alexandria (VA): CNA Corporation; 2003.
19. Guttmacher Institute. Medicaid family planning eligibility expansions; state policies in brief. 2015. Available at: http://www.guttmacher.org/statecenter/spibs/spib_SMFPE.pdf. Accessed May 10, 2015.
20. Center on Budget Policy and Priorities. How health reform's medicaid expansion will impact state budgets. Available at: http://www.cbpp.org/research/how-health-reforms-medicaid-expansion-will-impact-state-budgets. Accessed May 2, 2015.
21. Pace LE, Dusetzina SB, Fendrick AM, et al. The impact of out-of-pocket costs on the use of intrauterine contraception among women with employer-sponsored insurance. Med Care 2013;51:959–63.
22. Postlethwaite D, Trussell J, Zoolakis A, et al. A comparison of contraceptive procurement pre- and post-benefit change. Contraception 2007;76:360–5.
23. Secura GM, Allsworth JE, Madden T, et al. The Contraceptive CHOICE Project: reducing barriers to long-acting reversible contraception. Am J Obstet Gynecol 2010;203:115.e1–7.
24. Peipert JF, Madden T, Allsworth JE, et al. Preventing unintended pregnancies by providing no-cost contraception. Obstet Gynecol 2012;120:1291.
25. Trussell J. Contraceptive failure in the United States. Contraception 2004;70:89–96.
26. Winner B, Peipert JF, Zhao Q, et al. Effectiveness of long-acting reversible contraception. N Engl J Med 2012;366:1998–2007.

27. Trussell J, Henry N, Hassan F, et al. Burden of unintended pregnancy in the United States: potential savings with increased use of long-acting reversible contraception. Contraception 2013;87:154–61.

28. Sonfield A, Tapales A, Jones RK, et al. Impact of the federal contraceptive coverage guarantee on out-of-pocket payments for contraceptives: 2014 update. Contraception 2015;91:44–8.

29. IMS Institute of Healthcare Informatics. Medicine use and the shifting costs of healthcare: a review of the use of medicines in the United States in 2013. 2014. Available at: http://www.imshealth.com/deployedfiles/imshealth/Global/Content/Corporate/IMS%20Health%20Institute/Reports/Secure/IIHI_US_Use_of_Meds_for_2013.pdf. Accessed April 27, 2015.

30. The Henry J Kaiser Foundation. Status of state action on the medicaid expansion decision. 2015. Available at: http://kff.org/health-reform/state-indicator/state-activity-around-expanding-medicaid-under-the-affordable-care-act/. Accessed on July 13, 2015.

31. The Henry J Kaiser Foundation. A closer look at the impact of state decisions not to expand Medicaid on coverage for uninsured adults. Available at: http://kff.org/health-reform/state-indicator/state-activity-around-expanding-medicaid-under-the-affordable-care-act/. Accessed on April 29, 2015.

32. Garfield R, Damico A, Stephens J, et al. The coverage gap: uninsured poor adults in states that do not expand Medicaid–an update. Chicago (IL): Kaiser Family Foundation; 2014.

33. Sonfield A, Frost JJ, Gold RB. Estimating the impact of expanding Medicaid eligibility for family planning services: 2011 update. New York: Guttmacher Institute; 2011. p. 38.

34. The Henry J Kasier Foundation. Grandfathering explained. 2011. Available at: http://kff.org/search/?s=grandfathering+explained. Accessed May 1, 2015.

35. The Kaiser Family Foundation and Health Research and Educational Trust. Employer Health Benefits 2014 Annual Survey. 2014. Available at: http://kff.org/health-costs/report/2014-employer-health-benefits-survey/. Accessed April 29, 2015.

36. Sonfield A. Implementing the federal contraceptive coverage guarantee: progress and prospects. Guttmacher Policy Rev 2013;16:8–12.

37. FDA. Birth control guide. Available at: http://www.fda.gov/downloads/For Consumers/ByAudience/ForWomen/FreePublications/UCM356451.pdf. Accessed May 1, 2015.

38. Sobel L, Salganicoff A, Kurani N. Coverage of contraceptive services: a review of health insurance plans in five states. Chicago (IL): Henry J. Kaiser Family Foundation; 2015.

39. Centers for Medicare and Medicaid Services. FAQs about the Affordable Care Act Implementation (Part XXVI). Department of Health and Human Services, 2015. Available at: http://www.cms.gov/CCIIO/Resources/Fact-Sheets-and-FAQs/Downloads/aca_implementation_faqs26.pdf. Accessed May 1, 2015.

40. Perkins J, Singh D. ACA implementation: the court challenges continue. Ann Health Law 2014;23:200–28.

41. American Civil Liberties Union. Challenges to the Federal Contraceptive Rule. 2015. Available at: https://www.aclu.org/challenges-federal-contraceptive-coverage-rule. Accessed May 1, 2015.

42. NFIB v Sebelius. 567_U.S. (2012), 132 S. Ct.2566.

43. King v Burwell. 576_U.S. (2015), 14–114.

44. Health and Human Services. Coverage of certain preventive services under the Affordable Care Act - final rules. 45 CFR 147131. Federal Register. 2013-15866. Washington, DC: Government Publishing Office; 2013.

45. Guttmacher Institute. New rules detail compromise for contraceptive coverage guarantee 2013. Available at: http://www.guttmacher.org/media/inthenews/2013/07/01/. Accessed May 1, 2015.

46. Health and Human Services. Exemption and accommodations in connection with coverage of preventive health services. I45 CFR 147131. Federal Register. Washington, DC: Government Publishing Office; 2013.

47. Wheaton College vs Burwell. 573_US. 2014.

48. Moniz MH, Davis MM, Chang T. Attitudes about mandated coverage of birth control medication and other health benefits in a US national sample. JAMA 2014; 311:2539–41.

49. Patton EW, Hall KS, Dalton VK. How does religious affiliation affect women's attitudes toward reproductive health policy? Implications for the Affordable Care Act. Contraception 2015;91(6):513–9.

Over-the-Counter Access to Oral Contraceptives

Daniel Grossman, MD[a,b,*]

KEYWORDS

- Oral contraceptives • Over the counter • Access • Insurance coverage
- Prescription • Cost

KEY POINTS

- US women are very interested in being able to access oral contraceptives without a prescription.
- Women can accurately identify contraindications to use of oral contraceptives using simple checklists.
- In one study, continuation of oral contraceptives was significantly higher among over-the-counter users compared with women obtaining pills by prescription.
- Full insurance coverage of over-the-counter contraception would lead to more women using the product and a greater reduction in unintended pregnancy.

INTRODUCTION

Unintended pregnancy in the United States has remained persistently high over the past two decades, accounting for about half of all pregnancies.[1] A variety of factors contribute to nonuse of contraception, gaps in use, and early discontinuation, all of which put women at risk of unintended pregnancy. For some women, side effects, both experienced and feared, lead them to not use or stop using a method, whereas others just do not like the available methods. But other women report difficulties accessing contraception, including challenges getting a prescription or a method and problems paying for a method. In one study exploring gaps in use, 40% reported problems accessing or using methods.[2] In another study from a nationally representative sample, 30% of women who had ever tried to obtain a prescription for hormonal contraception reported difficulties obtaining the prescription or refills.[3]

The high cost of contraception has recently been addressed by the contraceptive coverage guarantee under the Affordable Care Act, which mandates that most private

This work was supported by a grant from the William and Flora Hewlett Foundation (Grant number 2012-7908).
[a] Ibis Reproductive Health, 1330 Broadway, Suite 1100, Oakland, CA 94612, USA; [b] Department of Obstetrics, Gynecology and Reproductive Sciences, Bixby Center for Global Reproductive Health, University of California, San Francisco, 1001 Potrero Avenue, San Francisco, CA 94110, USA
* Ibis Reproductive Health, 1330 Broadway, Suite 1100, Oakland, CA 94612.
E-mail address: DGrossman@ibisreproductivehealth.org

insurances cover methods approved by the Food and Drug Administration (FDA) without cost sharing, such as copayments or deductibles.[4] But the prescription requirement may be another barrier to use that is no longer medically necessary, and removing this obstacle could be an additional strategy to reduce unintended pregnancy.

At first glance, it seems likely that oral contraceptives (OCs) meet the FDA's criteria to be made available without a prescription. OCs have no significant toxicity if overdosed, and they are not addictive. Women themselves determine if they are at risk of unintended pregnancy, essentially self-diagnosing the condition for appropriate use of the product. The FDA will also want to see that women can safely take the medication without a clinician's screening, and take the medication as indicated over time without a clinician's explanation. This article reviews the evidence indicating whether OCs meet these criteria, and women's interest in an over-the-counter (OTC) pill and several policy issues related to a change in status for OCs.

WOMEN'S INTEREST IN ACCESS TO HORMONAL CONTRACEPTION WITHOUT A PRESCRIPTION

The American College of Obstetricians and Gynecologists commissioned a national survey in 1993 to measure women's attitudes toward OCs.[5] In general, women thought the pill was less effective and more dangerous than it truly is, and 86% said OCs are not safe enough to buy OTC without seeing a physician first. Another survey was performed in 1995 at one college among female students, and 65% said OCs should not be available OTC.[6] In the 20 years since these studies were performed, levonorgestrel emergency contraception products have become available OTC, and not surprisingly, women's opinions have changed.

In 2004 a nationally representative telephone survey explored women's interest in pharmacy access to hormonal contraception.[7] In this survey of 811 US women (aged 18–44), 68% of women reported they would start the pill, patch, or vaginal ring if it were available directly in a pharmacy with screening by a pharmacist. African American and Latina women were more than twice as likely as white women to express interest in pharmacy access. Interest was also higher among low-income women and uninsured women. In addition, 41% of all women not currently using any contraception, and 47% of uninsured women and 40% of low-income women not currently using hormonal contraception, said they would begin using a hormonal method if it were available from pharmacies without a prescription.

Another survey from 2006 of 601 unsterilized women in El Paso, Texas, who were not currently using hormonal contraception or the intrauterine device (IUD) explored women's interest in obtaining OCs OTC in the United States.[8] A total of 60% said they would be more likely to use OCs if the pill were available OTC in the United States. In regression analysis, women not currently using a contraceptive method were more likely than users of nonhormonal methods to say they might use the pill if available OTC (adjusted odds ratio, 1.54; $P<.05$).

Another nationally representative survey in 2011 explored this topic with 2046 women aged 18 to 44 years who were considered at risk of unintended pregnancy.[9] Overall, 62% reported being strongly or somewhat in favor of OCs being available OTC, and 37% of respondents said they were likely to use an OTC OC if one were available. Younger women and those with private or no insurance were significantly more likely to report being likely to use a future OTC OC, as were current pill users. However, 33% of women currently using a less effective birth control method (like condoms alone) and 28% of women using no method said they were very or somewhat likely to start using the pill if it were available OTC.[9]

Qualitative research has also explored interest in OTC access to OCs with low-income women in Boston in 2007 to 2009.[10] Most participants supported OTC access to OCs; however, participants raised concerns about the cost of OTC OCs and the safety of use for minors, first-time pill users, and women with certain medical conditions.

In contrast to the United States, women in most countries of the world are already able to access OCs without a prescription (**Fig. 1**).[11] In 35 countries, OCs are legally available OTC, and in another 11 countries, they are available without a prescription after a woman is screened for eligibility by a trained pharmacy staff person. In an additional 56 countries, OCs are available informally without a prescription despite that they should require one. Only 45 of 147 countries surveyed require a prescription to obtain OCs.

EVIDENCE REGARDING THE SAFETY AND EFFECTIVENESS OF OVER-THE-COUNTER ACCESS TO ORAL CONTRACEPTIVES

A great deal of evidence has established the safety of OCs and a host of noncontraceptive benefits of the medication, including prevention of ovarian and uterine cancer.[12,13] Although rare complications, such as myocardial infarction, stroke, and venous thromboembolism, have been associated with OC use, certain conditions have been identified that increase the risk of these adverse events while using OCs.[14] The US Centers for Disease Control and Prevention developed the Medical Eligibility Criteria for Contraceptive Use based on a similar document issued by the World Health Organization.[15] The Medical Eligibility Criteria lists various conditions, including use of certain medications, and indicates whether a woman with the condition is eligible for different contraceptives using four different categories.

Little research has documented the prevalence of these contraindications in the general public. One study of a sample of women aged 18 to 49 in El Paso, Texas, found that 39% of women had at least one relative or absolute contraindication to

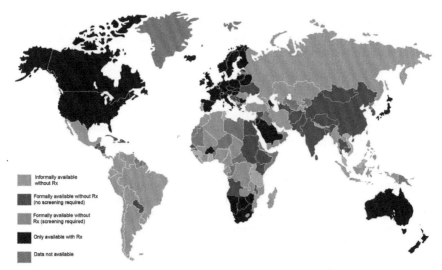

Fig. 1. Prescription requirements for oral contraceptives worldwide. (*Courtesy of* Ibis Reproductive Health and the Oral Contraceptives Over-the-Counter Working Group.)

combined hormonal contraception.[16] The most common contraindications were hypertension and migraine headache with aura. Less than 2% had a contraindication to progestin-only pills (POPs).[17] Other studies with women seeking contraception have found a much lower prevalence of contraindications to combined hormonal contraception.[18,19]

Studies have demonstrated that women can accurately self-identify these contraindications using a simple checklist. A study in Washington State found agreement between women's self-assessment of contraindications and the assessment of a clinician in 96% of cases (N = 399).[18] In the previously mentioned study from El Paso,[16] a self-screening checklist was found to have the following measures of accuracy:

- Sensitivity, 83.2% (95% confidence interval [CI], 79.5%–86.3%)
- Specificity, 88.8% (95% CI, 86.3%–90.9%)
- Positive predictive value, 82.8% (95% CI, 79.2%–86.0%)
- Negative predictive value, 89.0% (95% CI, 86.6%–91.1%)

Although the checklist performed well, 7% of women thought they were eligible for combined OCs (COCs) but were found to be ineligible by a nurse practitioner, generally because of unrecognized hypertension. A similar proportion of women thought they were ineligible because of severe headaches, but the nurse practitioner did not judge them to have the true contraindication of migraine with aura. The checklist was even more accurate to identify contraindications to POPs, with a negative predictive value of 99.6% (95% CI, 99.0%–99.8%).[17]

Given that there are fewer and rarer contraindications to the progestin-only formulation compared with COCs, it is likely that the first OTC OC in the United States will be a POP. This would also be a smaller leap from levonorgestrel emergency contraception, another progestin-only formulation, which has already been approved by the FDA for OTC sale.

Despite this evidence, the FDA will still require a company to perform specific research with the product it proposes to make available OTC. In particular, the company will have to develop a simple Drug Facts OTC label for the product and demonstrate that women can read and understand the key messages in the label (known as a label comprehension study). They will also have to perform a self-selection study demonstrating that women can use the label to accurately determine whether the product is appropriate for them.

EVIDENCE REGARDING ONGOING USE OF ORAL CONTRACEPTIVES IN AN OVER-THE-COUNTER ENVIRONMENT

Even in the current system where a prescription is required, adherence to OCs is far from perfect. One study using an electronic device to measure adherence found that one third of pill users missed three or more pills in a given cycle.[20] One-year continuation of OCs is reported to be 67%.[21]

No research has specifically documented the effectiveness of OCs in an OTC environment, although two studies have explored continuation of OCs in settings where they are available without a prescription. One study from Kuwait, where pills are available OTC, found that continuation was similar among women obtaining them without a prescription compared with those who consulted a physician.[22] In another study from El Paso, Texas, we compared women living in Texas who obtained OCs OTC in Mexican pharmacies across the border (N = 514) with women living in Texas who obtained pills by prescription in public clinics (N = 532).[23] In a multivariable analysis, discontinuation was significantly higher for women who obtained pills by prescription compared with the OTC users (hazard ratio, 1.6; 95% CI, 1.1–2.3).

Before approving an OC product for sale without a prescription, the FDA will require the pharmaceutical company to perform an actual use study to demonstrate that women can take the product appropriately over time. Although it is unclear exactly what the actual use study will require, it is likely to focus on adherence to the instructions for use over time, including taking the pill daily at the same time, taking appropriate measures in case of a missed pill, and continuation.

ADDITIONAL AREAS OF CONCERN RELATED TO A FUTURE OVER-THE-COUNTER ORAL CONTRACEPTIVE

Despite their strong support for OTC access to OCs, women have also expressed concerns. In addition to safety, these concerns have primarily focused on the cost of an OTC pill, whether women will continue to obtain recommended preventive screening, and whether OTC pills should be restricted to adults only. Clinicians have articulated similar concerns, as well as worries that the effort to make pills available OTC will undermine promotion of long-acting reversible contraception (LARC), and apprehension surrounding the selection of POPs to be the first OTC OC.

Cost and Insurance Coverage

When levonorgestrel emergency contraception became available OTC, the retail price was as high as $60, which has only recently begun to decrease.[24] This experience has brought the issue of price to the forefront of the debate about removing the prescription requirement for daily OCs. In a nationally representative survey of adult women at risk of unintended pregnancy conducted in 2011, among those interested in using an OTC OC, the average maximum price they were willing to pay for it was $20 per cycle; only 12% were willing to pay more than $30.[9] Of note, these data were collected before the contraceptive coverage guarantee under the Affordable Care Act went into effect. This provision requires most private insurances to cover FDA-approved contraceptive methods without cost sharing, such as copayments or deductibles. A recent study found that 67% of OC users with private insurance paid nothing out of pocket for their contraceptives.[25]

Although it is true that insurance has traditionally not covered OTC medications, more and more insurances are covering at least some nonprescription medicines.[26] Under the Women's Preventive Services Guidelines of the Affordable Care Act, OTC contraceptives that are FDA-approved and used by women also must be covered by insurance without cost sharing.[27] However, insurers may require a prescription to trigger such coverage, which obviously undermines any improvement in access afforded by making a method available OTC. Several state Medicaid programs cover OTC emergency contraception without requiring a prescription, providing a model for such coverage that could be expanded in others settings.[26]

A recent cost modeling analysis of a potential OTC OC product found that use among low-income women would be highest and the estimated reduction in unintended pregnancy would be greatest (7%–25%) if such pills were fully covered by insurance without cost sharing.[28] Full coverage would also be cost effective for insurances because of the savings associated with averting unwanted births.[28]

Adolescents and Over-the-Counter Access to a Future Oral Contraceptive

Perhaps the most controversial aspect of the OTC switch for levonorgestrel emergency contraception was whether adolescents should be able to access the product without a prescription. A concern that is often voiced by the public is that OTC access to contraception will result in teenagers having more unprotected sex or having sex at an earlier age.[9] However, studies have shown that free access to emergency contraception does not result in increased sexual risk-taking among adolescents.[29]

A growing body of evidence indicates that teenagers are interested in using OTC OCs. In a study of women obtaining abortion in six cities across the United States, 47% of clients aged 15 to 17 years old said they were likely to use an OTC OC if one were available.[30] In another online survey of female adolescents aged 14 to 17 years old, 61% reported they were likely to use a future OTC pill.[31]

Only 26% of adult women surveyed thought that an OTC OC should be restricted to women age 18 and older; 28% were against an age restriction, and 46% were unsure.[32] From a medical perspective, there is no reason to restrict OTC access to OCs to adults, but the FDA will likely require data from adolescent participants in the label comprehension, self-selection, and actual use studies to determine whether or not an age restriction is appropriate.

Preventive Screening

Another concern expressed by women and some clinicians is that women may not get recommended screening for cervical cancer or sexually transmitted infections if they do not have to come to a clinic to obtain hormonal contraception.[9] Despite a long-standing recommendation not to hold women's contraception hostage to force them to obtain such screening,[33] some providers continue to do so.[34] Ironically, in the discussion about promoting LARC methods, one seldom hears a concern that women will not get recommended screening after placement of a copper IUD, even though the method may last as long as 12 years.

Evidence from the cohort study in El Paso mentioned previously indicates that failure to obtain preventive services should not be a serious concern. Among women obtaining OCs by prescription, 99% had obtained cervical cancer screening within the prior 3 years, compared with 91% of OTC pill users.[35] Although these differences were significant, the proportions in both groups were higher than the national average of 85%. The most common reason women gave for not having had recent screening for cervical cancer was that it was too expensive, and many of the OTC users had obtained their last Pap smear in Mexico. Similar results were observed for sexually transmitted infection screening and clinical breast examinations.

Lost Opportunity to Counsel About Long-Acting Reversible Contraception Methods

Some clinicians have voiced concerns that making OCs available OTC will promote a method less effective than contraceptive implants and IUDs and that elimination of the clinical encounter will reduce opportunities to counsel about LARC.[36] Although there may be some truth in this, our current model for providing contraception also does not optimize opportunities for a discussion of LARC. One study of more than 1300 young women getting family planning services at clinics in the San Francisco Bay area in 2005 to 2007 found that only 10% reported that their provider discussed the IUD.[37]

There is also evidence that women seeking OCs in a pharmacy without a prescription are not interested in LARC. In a pilot study in London, England, pharmacists were trained to screen women for medical eligibility and provide OCs. They were also trained to counsel all women about LARC methods and to refer those who were interested. Of 741 consultations over a period of 21 months, only 9 women (1.2%) were referred for LARC.[38] When an OTC OC is actually launched, it will be important to couple this with an informational campaign about all contraceptive methods, including LARC.

Lack of Familiarity with Progestin-Only Pills

Only about 4% of OC users in the United States use POPs, and these are primarily postpartum women and older women with medical contraindications to COCs.[39] If a POP is the first OC to become available OTC, women will need to be informed about the differences between this formulation and COCs, including

- Pills are taken daily without a hormone-free period at the end of the cycle.
- Although there is limited published data supporting this recommendation, the labeling for POPs says that if a pill is taken more than 3 hours late, women must either abstain or use a barrier method of contraception until they are back on the pill for 48 hours.
- Breakthrough bleeding is more common with POPs than with COCs.

Some physicians have a perception that POPs are less effective than COCs, but a recent Cochrane review comparing the efficacy of the two formulations found there was insufficient evidence to draw a conclusion regarding this outcome.[40] In the class labeling of OCs, the effectiveness of COCs and POPs is noted to be equivalent.[21]

PHARMACY ACCESS TO HORMONAL CONTRACEPTION

Another model to improve access to hormonal contraception involves pharmacist provision, also known as pharmacy access. Before emergency contraception became available OTC, this model allowed women to access the method in a pharmacy without a prescription. For hormonal contraception, women generally complete a questionnaire to identify contraindications, and then a trained pharmacist measures blood pressure and reviews the questionnaire. Depending on the setting and the level of training of the pharmacist, counseling is also provided about the different methods.

Pharmacy access to hormonal contraception has been most widely used in Washington State, where pharmacists have been able to provide the pill, patch, and ring through collaborative practice agreements with physicians. An evaluation of the model found that it was safe, effective, and feasible, and women were satisfied with the services.[41] Unfortunately, few insurers reimbursed pharmacists for their time, so women had to pay out of pocket for the screening and counseling, which ultimately limited the expansion of the model. Laws have recently been passed in California, Oregon and the District of Columbia that will allow pharmacists to provide hormonal contraception, and it will be interesting to see how access for women is improved in these settings.

The pharmacy access model is a promising strategy to reduce barriers to contraception. In particular, because a pharmacist generates a prescription for the method, women with insurance should be able to obtain coverage for birth control obtained in this way. A national survey of pharmacists found that most are interested in becoming more involved in providing hormonal contraception, although they were concerned about receiving adequate reimbursement.[42] Other concerns about the model include the need to establish such protocols in each state and provide training for the pharmacists. In addition, some pharmacists may refuse to provide hormonal contraception, as they have done with emergency contraception,[43] which would limit access.

SUPPORT FOR OVER-THE-COUNTER ACCESS TO ORAL CONTRACEPTIVE AMONG PROFESSIONAL MEDICAL AND NURSING GROUPS

A growing number of professional organizations have voiced their support for making OCs available OTC, and these are noted in **Table 1**.

Table 1	
Medical and nursing organizations that have expressed support for OTC access to OCs	
Organization	**Policy Statement**
American Academy of Family Physicians	Supports OTC access to OCs with insurance coverage[44]
American College of Nurse-Midwives	Signed on to the statement of purpose of the Oral Contraceptives Over-the-Counter Working Group[45]
American College of Obstetricians and Gynecologists	Supports OTC access to OCs with insurance coverage, noting that OTC access to OCs has the potential to reduce unintended pregnancy and that the benefits of OTC access outweigh the possible risks[46,47]
American Medical Association	Asks the FDA to encourage pharmaceutical companies to submit the necessary evidence that would support an OTC switch for an OC product[48]
American Public Health Association	Supports insurance coverage of OTC contraception without requiring a prescription[49]
Association of Reproductive Health Professionals	Signed on to the statement of purpose of the Oral Contraceptives Over-the-Counter Working Group[45]
National Association of Nurse Practitioners in Women's Health	Signed on to the statement of purpose of the Oral Contraceptives Over-the-Counter Working Group[45]
Society of General Internal Medicine Women's Health Task Force	Signed on to the statement of purpose of the Oral Contraceptives Over-the-Counter Working Group[45]
Women's Health Practice and Research Network of the American College of Clinical Pharmacy	Supports OTC access to OCs provided they are sold where a pharmacist is on duty and that there are mechanisms in place to cover OTC contraceptives through Medicaid[50]

Data from Refs.[44–50]

SUMMARY

Making OCs available OTC has the potential to dramatically change the way women obtain birth control and could lead to a significant reduction in unintended pregnancy in the United States. Although it is likely that a POP will be the first OC product to be made available OTC, it is hoped this will be an interim step leading to approval of an OTC COC product, and eventually other contraceptive methods.

It is critical that the move toward OTC availability address issues of access, including cost. If an OTC pill is priced too high, women with the most to gain from it will be unable to purchase it. Insurance coverage of OTC contraception makes sense from a public health and economic perspective and must be part of the policy agenda as more OTC methods become available. Manufacturers must also make an OTC OC product available at an accessible price for women without insurance, perhaps using tiered pricing. In addition, unless there is evidence indicating that adolescents are unable to use an OTC pill appropriately, approved products should not have age restrictions. This means that pharmaceutical companies must include adolescents in the studies that the FDA will require to consider making OCs available OTC.

Making the pill available OTC could also help to demedicalize contraception and make it more of a consumer product, which in turn may improve perceptions about the safety of birth control. By putting more effective contraception on the pharmacy and grocery store shelf, women could be empowered to take control of their reproductive health care and better plan their pregnancies.

REFERENCES

1. Finer LB, Zolna MR. Unintended pregnancy in the United States: incidence and disparities, 2006. Contraception 2011;84(5):478–85.
2. Frost JJ, Singh S, Finer LB. U.S. women's one-year contraceptive use patterns, 2004. Perspect Sex Reprod Health 2007;39(1):48–55.
3. Grindlay K, Grossman D. Prescription birth control access among a representative sample of US women at risk of unintended pregnancy. Contraception 2013;88: 452–3.
4. U.S. Department of Health and Human Services. Women's preventive services guidelines. Available at: http://www.hrsa.gov/womensguidelines/. Accessed June 21, 2015.
5. Murphy P, Kirkman A, Hale RW. A national survey of women's attitudes toward oral contraception and other forms of birth control. Womens Health Issues 1995;5(2): 94–9.
6. Forman SF, Emans SJ, Kelly L, et al. Attitudes of female college students toward over-the-counter availability of oral contraceptives. J Pediatr Adolesc Gynecol 1997;10(4):203–7.
7. Landau SC, Tapias MP, McGhee BT. Birth control within reach: a national survey on women's attitudes toward and interest in pharmacy access to hormonal contraception. Contraception 2006;74:463–70.
8. Grossman D, Fernández L, Hopkins K, et al. Perceptions of the safety of oral contraceptives among a predominantly Latina population in Texas. Contraception 2010;81(3):254–60.
9. Grossman D, Grindlay K, Li R, et al. Interest in over-the-counter access to oral contraceptives among women in the United States. Contraception 2013;88(4):544–52.
10. Dennis A, Grossman D. Barriers to contraception and interest in over-the-counter access among low-income women: a qualitative study. Perspect Sex Reprod Health 2012;44(2):84–91.
11. Grindlay K, Burns B, Grossman D. Prescription requirements and over-the-counter access to oral contraceptives: a global review. Contraception 2013;88(1):91–6.
12. Hannaford PC, Iversen L, Macfarlane TV, et al. Mortality among contraceptive pill users: cohort evidence from Royal College of General Practitioners' Oral Contraception Study. BMJ 2010;340:c927.
13. Havrilesky LJ, Moorman PG, Lowery WJ, et al. Oral contraceptive pills as primary prevention for ovarian cancer: a systematic review and meta-analysis. Obstet Gynecol 2013;122(1):139–47.
14. Schwingl PJ, Ory HW, Visness CM. Estimates of the risk of cardiovascular death attributable to low-dose oral contraceptives in the United States. Am J Obstet Gynecol 1999;180(1 Pt 1):241–9.
15. Centers for Disease Control and Prevention (CDC). U S. medical eligibility criteria for contraceptive use, 2010. MMWR Recomm Rep 2010;59(RR-4):1–86.
16. Grossman D, Fernandez L, Hopkins K, et al. Accuracy of self-screening for contraindications to combined oral contraceptive use. Obstet Gynecol 2008; 112(3):572–8.
17. White K, Potter JE, Hopkins K, et al. Contraindications to progestin-only oral contraceptive pills among reproductive-aged women. Contraception 2012; 86(3):199–203.

18. Shotorbani S, Miller L, Blough DK, et al. Agreement between women's and providers' assessment of hormonal contraceptive risk factors. Contraception 2006;73(5):501–6.

19. Xu H, Eisenberg DL, Madden T, et al. Medical contraindications in women seeking combined hormonal contraception. Am J Obstet Gynecol 2014;210(3):210.e1–5.

20. Potter L, Oakley D, de Leon-Wong E, et al. Measuring compliance among oral contraceptive users. Fam Plann Perspect 1996;28(4):154–8.

21. Trussell J. Contraceptive failure in the United States. Contraception 2011;83(5):397–404.

22. Shah MA, Shah NM, Al-Rahmani E, et al. Over-the-counter use of oral contraceptives in Kuwait. Int J Gynaecol Obstet 2001;73(3):243–51.

23. Potter JE, McKinnon S, Hopkins K, et al. Continuation of prescribed compared with over-the-counter oral contraceptives. Obstet Gynecol 2011;117(3):551–7.

24. American Society for Emergency Contraception. The cost of emergency contraception: results from a nationwide survey (July 2013). Available at: http://americansocietyforec.org/uploads/3/2/7/0/3270267/asecpricingreport.pdf. Accessed July 15, 2015.

25. Sonfield A, Tapales A, Jones RK, et al. Impact of the federal contraceptive coverage guarantee on out-of-pocket payments for contraceptives: 2014 update. Contraception 2015;91(1):44–8.

26. McIntosh J, Wahlin B, Grindlay K, et al. Insurance and access implications of an over-the-counter switch for a progestin-only pill. Perspect Sex Reprod Health 2013;45(3):164–9.

27. FAQs about Affordable Care Act implementation part XII. United States Department of Labor, Department of Health and Human Services, and Department of the Treasury. Available at: http://www.dol.gov/ebsa/faqs/faq-aca12.html. Accessed June 21, 2015.

28. Foster DG, Biggs MA, Phillips KA, et al. Potential public sector cost-savings from over-the-counter access to oral contraceptives. Contraception 2015;91(5):373–9.

29. Harper CC, Cheong M, Rocca CH, et al. The effect of increased access to emergency contraception among young adolescents. Obstet Gynecol 2005;106(3):483–91.

30. Grindlay K, Foster DG, Grossman D. Attitudes toward over-the-counter access to oral contraceptives among a sample of abortion clients in the United States. Perspect Sex Reprod Health 2014;46(2):83–9.

31. Manski R, Kottke M. A Survey of Teenagers' Attitudes Toward Moving Oral Contraceptives Over the Counter. Perspect Sex Reprod Health 2015.

32. Grindlay K, Grossman D. Women's perspectives on age restrictions for over-the-counter access to oral contraceptives. J Adolesc Health 2015;56(1):38–43.

33. Stewart FH, Harper CC, Ellertson CE, et al. Clinical breast and pelvic examination requirements for hormonal contraception: current practice vs evidence. JAMA 2001;285(17):2232–9.

34. Schwarz EB, Saint M, Gildengorin G, et al. Cervical cancer screening continues to limit provision of contraception. Contraception 2005;72(3):179–81.

35. Hopkins K, Grossman D, White K, et al. Reproductive health preventive screening among clinic vs. over-the-counter oral contraceptive users. Contraception 2012;86(4):376–82.

36. Jarvis S. Should the contraceptive pill be available without prescription? No. BMJ 2008;337:a3056.

37. Harper CC, Brown BA, Foster-Rosales A, et al. Hormonal contraceptive method choice among young, low-income women: how important is the provider? Patient Educ Couns 2010;81(3):349–54.

38. Parsons J, Adams C, Aziz N, et al. Evaluation of a community pharmacy delivered oral contraception service. J Fam Plann Reprod Health Care 2013;39(2):97–101.

39. Liang SY, Grossman D, Phillips KA. User characteristics and out-of-pocket expenditures for progestin-only versus combined oral contraceptives. Contraception 2012;86(6):666–72.

40. Grimes DA, Lopez LM, O'Brien PA, et al. Progestin-only pills for contraception. Cochrane Database Syst Rev 2013;(11):CD007541.

41. Gardner JS, Miller L, Downing DF, et al. Pharmacist prescribing of hormonal contraceptives: results of the Direct Access study. J Am Pharm Assoc (2003) 2008; 48(2):212–21, 5 p following 221.

42. Landau S, Besinque K, Chung F, et al. Pharmacist interest in and attitudes toward direct pharmacy access to hormonal contraception in the United States. J Am Pharm Assoc (2003) 2009;49(1):43–50.

43. Richman AR, Daley EM, Baldwin J, et al. The role of pharmacists and emergency contraception: are pharmacists' perceptions of emergency contraception predictive of their dispensing practices? Contraception 2012;86(4):370–5.

44. American Academy of Family Physicians. Over-the-counter oral contraceptives. Available at: http://www.aafp.org/about/policies/all/otc-oral-contraceptives.html. Accessed June 21, 2015.

45. Oral Contraceptives Over-the-Counter Working Group Statement of Purpose. Available at: http://ocsotc.org/?page_id=5. Accessed June 21, 2015.

46. Committee on Gynecologic Practice, American College of Obstetricians and Gynecologists. Committee opinion No 544: over-the-counter access to oral contraceptives. Obstet Gynecol 2012;120(6):1527–31.

47. Committee on Health Care for Underserved Women. Committee opinion no. 615: access to contraception. Obstet Gynecol 2015;125(1):250–5.

48. American Medical Association. D-75.995 Over-the-Counter Access to Oral Contraceptives. Available at: https://www.ama-assn.org/ssl3/ecomm/PolicyFinder Form.pl?site=www.ama-assn.org&;uri=%2fresources%2fhtml%2fPolicyFinder %2fpolicyfiles%2fDIR%2fD-75.995.HTM. Accessed June 21, 2015.

49. American Public Health Association. Improving Access to Over the Counter Contraception by Expanding Insurance Coverage. Available at: http://www.apha.org/ policies-and-advocacy/public-health-policy-statements/policy-database/2014/ 07/24/10/31/improving-access-to-over-the-counter-contraception-by-expanding-insurance-coverage. Accessed June 21, 2015.

50. McIntosh J, Rafie S, Wasik M, et al. Changing oral contraceptives from prescription to over-the-counter status: an opinion statement of the Women's Health Practice and Research Network of the American College of Clinical Pharmacy. Pharmacotherapy 2011;31(4):424–37.

Providing Contraception to Adolescents

Shandhini Raidoo, MD*, Bliss Kaneshiro, MD, MPH

KEYWORDS

- Adolescents • Teens • Contraception • Birth control
- Long-acting reversible contraception • Intrauterine device • Implant • Access

KEY POINTS

- Although rates are decreasing, unintended pregnancy continues to be a significant health care problem for adolescents.
- Long-acting reversible contraceptives are recommended for adolescents because they are highly effective, easy to use, and have few side effects.
- Education, cost, and access are important barriers that must be overcome when providing contraception for adolescents.

INTRODUCTION

Although adolescent pregnancy continues to represent a significant public health problem, pregnancy rates in adolescents are on the decline. In 1990, the pregnancy rate among 15- to 19-year-olds in the United States was 116.9 per 1000 women.[1] By 2010, this rate had dropped 51% to 57.4 per 1000 women.[1] The birth rate among adolescents in 2010 was 34.4 per 1000 women, the lowest since the peak of 61.8 per 1000 women in 1991. The abortion rate was 14.7 per 1000 women, the lowest since the peak of 43.5 in 1988.[1,2] Despite these encouraging statistics, the United States remains the developed country with the highest rate of teenage pregnancy.[3] Other developed countries report teen pregnancy rates as low as 8 per 1000 (Switzerland) and 14 per 1000 (Netherlands).[3]

Unintended pregnancy has significant costs for individuals and the health care system as a whole. Unintended pregnancy in adolescents costs the United States an estimated $9.4 billion in 2010.[4] Twenty-six percent of high school dropouts cite becoming a parent as the reason for dropping out, while one-third of adolescent women report

The authors have no conflicts to disclose.

Department of Obstetrics, Gynecology, and Women's Health, Kapiolani Medical Center for Women and Children, University of Hawaii John A. Burns School of Medicine, 1319 Punahou Street, Suite 824, Honolulu, HI 96826, USA

* Corresponding author.

E-mail address: sraidoo@hawaii.edu

pregnancy or parenting as the reason they did not complete high school.[5] Adolescents who drop out of high school are less likely to return to complete a high school diploma or General Educational Development, are more likely to be unemployed, and have lower incomes than their peers who complete high school.[5]

Most adolescents become sexually active during their teenage years, and providing them with effective contraception is vitally important. In the National Survey of Family Growth, the percentage of adolescents who had had sexual intercourse increased from 2% at age 12 to 71% by age 19 years.[6] Seventy-eight percent of females and 85% of males report using some form of contraception at first intercourse, with the majority (68% of females and 80% of males) using condoms the first time they have sex.[7] Use of contraception among adolescents has increased since 1995, with 86% of females and 93% of males reporting using any contraception at last intercourse.[6] Dual protection, the use of both condoms and more effective methods as protection against sexually transmitted infection (STI) and unwanted pregnancy, is the ideal contraceptive practice, but is reported by only 20% of sexually active females and 34% of sexually active males.[6]

Women who use long-acting reversible contraception (LARC) such as intrauterine devices (IUDs) and implants have lower rates of unintended pregnancy. Other methods are less effective because they depend highly on user compliance. The 18% of women who use contraception inconsistently account for 41% of the total unintended pregnancies.[8,9] Though cited as first-line contraceptive methods for adolescents, implants and IUDs are used by only 4.5% of adolescent women.[10]

ADOLESCENT HEALTH
Cognitive Development

Adolescence is a period of transition from childhood to adulthood consisting of rapid physical and cognitive change. The frontal lobes, largely responsible for higher-order functions such as decision making, prioritization, and abstract thinking, undergo significant development during puberty.[11] The prefrontal cortex is not fully developed until age 25 years, and is responsible for organization, impulse control, and strategy formation.[11] This developing ability for decision making and abstract thinking presents a challenge when caring for adolescents, and is an important consideration when counseling adolescents about high-risk behavior and risk reduction.

High-Risk Behavior

Experimentation with substance use during adolescence can alter inhibitions and render adolescents more susceptible to unwanted sexual activity. The 2013 Youth Risk Behavior Surveillance reported that 22.4% of adolescents had used drugs or alcohol before their last sexual intercourse.[12] Adolescent women are at increased risk for physical dating violence compared with adult women, and 13% of adolescent women reported physical violence from a partner within the past 12 months while 14.4% of adolescent women reported sexual dating violence, or being forced to engage in sexual behavior against their will.[12]

THE ADOLESCENT REPRODUCTIVE HEALTH VISIT

The American College of Obstetricians and Gynecologists (ACOG) recommends an initial reproductive health visit at age 13 to 15 years to establish a patient-provider relationship and to begin assessment of risk behaviors and counseling on risk reduction.[13] The pelvic examination is a concern for many adolescents, and they should be informed that this examination is not required unless they have specific complaints such as abnormal discharge, pelvic or abdominal pain, or abnormal bleeding.[13]

Confidentiality

Adolescents are learning to assert their independence and participate in health care decision making. The Society for Adolescent Medicine recommends establishing a policy of confidentiality with the adolescent patient and her parent or guardian at the start of a health care visit.[14] Restrictions on confidentiality, including the need to report suspected abuse, suicidality or homicidality, and certain diseases should be disclosed.[13] Establishing a trusting patient-provider relationship with adolescents is key to allowing open, candid communication, which facilitates an accurate assessment of the patient's risks and behaviors. A portion of the visit should be conducted without the parent or guardian being present so that topics such as sexual behavior and use of alcohol or drugs can be assessed.[14]

Sexually Transmitted Infections

Almost 50% (9.1 million) of the 18.9 million STIs diagnosed in the United States each year are diagnosed in young people aged 15 to 24 years.[15] During the reproductive health visit, the prevention of STIs with barrier contraception should be discussed.[13] If adolescents are sexually active, they should be encouraged to have testing for STIs. Testing for gonorrhea and chlamydia can be accomplished with nucleic acid amplification testing from urine, cervical sample, or a self-collected vaginal swab, whereas testing for human immunodeficiency virus (HIV), syphilis, and hepatitis requires blood sampling. Sexually active women younger than 25 years should undergo testing annually for gonorrhea and chlamydia, and be tested for HIV at least once, with more frequent STI testing in adolescents who are determined to be at higher risk for infection.[16]

Sexual Behavior and Contraception

A discussion on reproduction, sexual activity, and pregnancy prevention can be tailored to the adolescent's needs. Issues of consent, related risk behaviors (drug and alcohol use), and dating violence[13] should also be discussed. Adolescents should be counseled on the risks associated with both noncoital sexual activity and penile-vaginal intercourse.[17] Contraceptive counseling should be comprehensive, with a focus on efficacy and ease of use.[18] Many forms of hormonal contraception result in alterations of bleeding patterns that can be of concern to adolescents, who may have concrete expectations of menstruation.[19] Counseling on anticipated side effects may decrease the rates of dissatisfaction and discontinuation.[20]

CONTRACEPTIVE OPTIONS IN ADOLESCENTS
Long-Acting Reversible Contraception

LARC methods have high efficacy and require no action on the part of the adolescent after placement or insertion, resulting in perfect and typical use rates that closely approximate each other.[18] Among adolescents, satisfaction with LARC is high and discontinuation is low.[21] Because of these qualities, ACOG and the American Academy of Pediatrics have endorsed LARC as a first-line method for pregnancy prevention among adolescents.[18,22] In 2002, LARC use in the United States among adolescents using contraception was 0.3%, and this increased to 4.5% in 2009.[10] In federally funded Title X clinic sites the use of IUDs among adolescents increased from 0.4% to 2.8%, and the use of implants increased from 0.04% to 4.3% from 2005 to 2013.[23] Although LARC use has increased dramatically, it is still underutilized in adolescents.

Etonogestrel Implant

The etonogestrel implant is the most effective form of contraception, with a perfect and typical use failure rate of 0.05%.[24] The etonogestrel implant is approved for 3 years of use by the Food and Drug Administration (FDA), but has been demonstrated to continue to be effective for up to 5 years of use, with serum levels of etonogestrel well above the therapeutic threshold during this time interval.[25]

Bleeding patterns will change with the etonogestrel implant, and adolescents should be thoroughly counseled about expected bleeding patterns with implant use. A study documenting bleeding patterns with the etonogestrel implant noted that 22.4% of women will experience amenorrhea, 33.6% infrequent bleeding, 17.7% prolonged bleeding, and 6.7% frequent bleeding.[26] The bleeding patterns demonstrated during the first 3 months of use are predictive of the patterns that will occur for the duration of use.[26] A study on menstrual irregularities in adolescents with the etonogestrel implant demonstrated a discontinuation rate of 22.4% because of abnormal bleeding.[27] Adolescents should be reassured that the implant continues to be highly effective regardless of changes in bleeding pattern. Amenorrhea, irregular bleeding, and spotting or prolonged bleeding do not indicate a problem with the implant. Although a change in bleeding is expected with implant use, patients presenting with new-onset changes in bleeding and a history or symptoms concerning for cervicitis should be tested for STIs.[28]

Levonorgestrel Intrauterine Devices

There are currently 3 levonorgestrel IUDs available in the United States: the 13.5-mg levonorgestrel IUD and 2 types of 52-mg levonorgestrel IUDs.[29] The 13.5-mg IUD is marketed for use in nulliparous women and adolescents because of its smaller size and narrower inserter. A randomized controlled trial demonstrated high acceptability rates with both types of levonorgestrel IUDs, although insertion was slightly less painful and unscheduled bleeding was more common with the 13.5-mg levonorgestrel IUD.[30]

Perfect use and typical use failure rates for the levonorgestrel IUD are identical, at 0.2%.[24] Adolescents should be counseled about expected changes in bleeding patterns. One-third of women using the 52-mg levonorgestrel IUD experience oligomenorrhea immediately following insertion, and 70% of women experience oligomenorrhea or amenorrhea after 2 years of use.[31] Six percent of women using the 13.5-mg levonorgestrel IUD will experience oligomenorrhea immediately following insertion, and less than 50% of women experience oligomenorrhea or amenorrhea after 2 years of use.[30] Because of these favorable changes in bleeding patterns, the levonorgestrel IUD is commonly used in adolescents for the treatment of menorrhagia, dysmenorrhea, and inherited bleeding disorders.[32–34]

Copper Intrauterine Device

The copper IUD currently in use in the United States is the TCu380A IUD, which has a total exposed copper area of 380 mm^2.[35] Perfect use failure rate is 0.6% and typical use failure rate is 0.8% in the first year of use.[24] The copper IUD is the only IUD currently available in the United States with no hormonal component, and may be attractive to adolescents who desire a nonhormonal method. The copper IUD is approved for use for up to 10 years, although research indicates that it remains effective for up to 12 years.[29] The release of copper ions from the IUD causes an inflammatory reaction that limits the entrance of sperm into the uterus, and it has a sterile foreign-body effect on the uterine cavity that creates a toxic environment for sperm.[36,37] Copper-containing IUDs are contraindicated in patients with Wilson disease and severe anemia of unexplained origin.[38]

The most common side effects are an increase in menstrual bleeding over the first 1 to 3 months, after which the amount of bleeding remains stable for the duration of use. Despite the heavier bleeding, no negative effect on anemia-related iron parameters has been noted.[39] Discontinuation rates at 6, 13, and 25 months are 8%, 13.8%, and 21.7%, respectively.[40] Adolescents who elect for a copper IUD cite a desire for continued menses and a nonhormonal method, and the most common reason for discontinuation among adolescents is bleeding irregularities.[41]

An additional benefit of the copper IUD is its utility for emergency contraception. It is highly effective, with a pregnancy rate of 0.1% to 0.2% if inserted within 120 hours of unprotected intercourse, and is a highly effective option for women who desire a long-term form of contraception.[42,43]

Special Considerations for Use of Intrauterine Devices Among Adolescents

IUD expulsion rates for nulliparous women are lower than those in multiparous women, although rates of expulsion are slightly higher (5%–18%) among women 14 to 19 years of age compared with women older than 19 (3%–5%).[44,45] Rates of perforation with insertion are estimated to be very low, approximately 1 to 2 per 1000, and do not vary based on patient age.[46]

Adolescents have rates of pain with IUD insertion similar to those in adult women,[47] but higher rates of pain with insertion have been noted in nulliparous women than in multiparous women.[47–49] Studies have not clearly identified any one method that is effective for pain management at the time of insertion, so any interventions should be tailored to the individual's needs.[18] Studies on the use of cervical lidocaine for insertion have demonstrated a small effect on decreasing pain, although results are limited.[18,50,51] No difference in pain scores has been noted with the use of prophylactic ibuprofen for insertion.[48,49] Studies on the use of misoprostol for insertion demonstrate no increase in ease of insertion and no decrease in patient-reported pain.[52,53]

Sexually Transmitted Infection Testing and Pelvic Inflammatory Disease

STI screening before IUD insertion should be done in accordance with the current STI testing guidelines.[54] Patients who require screening can be tested at the time of insertion and, if positive, treated at the time of the result without removal of the IUD.[55] If active evidence of cervicitis is evident at the time of insertion, IUD placement should be deferred until the patient has been treated.[56] Despite concerns, the rate of pelvic inflammatory disease is low: 0% to 2% if there is no infection present at the time of insertion, and 0% to 5% if there is a documented infection.[57] No antibiotic prophylaxis is recommended for IUD insertion.[18]

Postpregnancy Insertion

Implants and IUDs can be inserted immediately after a suction aspiration for abortion or miscarriage and after vaginal and cesarean delivery, with acceptable rates of continuation and satisfaction.[58] Access to immediate postpregnancy insertion is especially important for adolescents who are more motivated to prevent pregnancy following an abortion or a delivery.[18] Although rates of expulsion are higher following postpregnancy insertion than after interval insertion, rates of continuation at 6 months are higher when compared with women who were planning delayed placement, as many patients do not return for insertion.[58,59]

Progestin-Only Methods

Depot medroxyprogesterone acetate

Depot medroxyprogesterone acetate (DMPA) is given in an intramuscular injection of 150 mg or a subcutaneous formulation of 104 mg every 3 months. The typical use failure rate is 6%, which is largely a result of user failure to return for repeat injection given that perfect use failure rates are estimated to be 0.2%.[24] Twenty percent of adolescents report ever using DMPA for contraception, whereas 3% report using it as their current contraceptive method.[60]

The most common side effect is irregular bleeding, which is more common during the first 3 to 9 months of use.[61] The amenorrhea rate after 12 months of use is greater than 50%.[62] Rates of discontinuation are high among adolescents; almost half will discontinue DMPA within 6 months of initiation.[61,63] The most common reasons for discontinuation among adolescents are irregular bleeding and weight gain.[61,63]

DMPA use is associated with a small increase in weight gain, which is more pronounced in obese adolescent girls than in their nonobese counterparts.[64,65] Although concerns have been raised about the effect of DMPA on bone mineral density (BMD), no evidence of increased fracture risk in adolescents with long-term DMPA use has been noted.[66] The potential risk of temporarily decreased BMD should not prevent the use of this effective form of contraception in adolescents, and the duration of use should not be limited in adolescents and women without additional risk factors for fractures.[67]

Progestin-only pills

Progestin-only pills (POPs) consist of a progestin component in a daily oral tablet, and functions to thicken cervical mucus to limit the penetration of sperm, inhibiting ovulation in up to 60% of women.[36] POPs are less effective than other progestin-only methods of contraception. Whereas POPs will prevent more pregnancies in comparison with no method, they are not highly recommended in adolescents because of the need for daily compliance.[60] Only 0.4% of women use POPs, most of whom are postpartum or lactating.[68]

Combined Hormonal Contraception

Combined hormonal contraception (CHC) includes pills, patch, and rings that contain an estrogen component and a progestin component. All forms of CHC have similar failure rates of 9% with typical use.[24]

Noncontraceptive benefits

CHC is often initiated in adolescents for its noncontraceptive benefits including improvements in dysmenorrhea, menorrhagia, acne, iron deficiency anemia, menstrual migraines, and menstrual irregularities.[69,70] Many adolescents may initiate the use of CHC, typically combined with oral contraceptives, for menorrhagia or dysmenorrhea soon after menarche, and often before becoming sexually active.[71]

Side effects

The most common side effect of CHC is irregular bleeding, which occurs more commonly in the first 3 cycles following initiation and then decreases with increased duration of use.[70] Although many adolescents are concerned about weight gain with the use of CHC, a Cochrane systematic review on weight gain with various forms of CHC reported no demonstrable change in weight.[72] Estrogen-containing contraceptives are associated with a 2- to 6-fold increase in the rate of venous thromboembolism (VTE),[70] although it should be noted that these rates remain lower than the risk of VTE with pregnancy.[73,74]

Combined oral contraceptives

Many different combined oral contraceptive (COC) formulations are available to patients. COCs are the most commonly used form of contraception among adolescents.[12] Fifty-six percent of adolescents report ever using COCs, and 15% report using them for contraception currently.[60] Adolescents who choose COCs as their method of contraception should be counseled on adherence to a daily schedule, as up to 52% of young women report missing at least 1 pill per month while 14% report missing more than 1 pill a month.[75] More than 50% of adolescents discontinue the use of COCs within 12 months, and most do so within the first 3 to 6 months of use.[76,77] The most common reason for discontinuation overall is irregular bleeding. Adolescents are also more likely to discontinue because of weight gain, although weight gain is not a side effect of CHC use.[77]

Contraceptive patch

The contraceptive patch consists of a transdermal adhesive patch applied to the skin and is replaced every 7 days for 3 weeks, followed by a patch-free interval of 3 to 7 days for a withdrawal bleed. The patch is associated with high rates of satisfaction in adolescents, although it has a higher rate of discontinuation in comparison with COCs.[78] The most common reasons for discontinuation among adolescents are cost, skin irritation, and detachment of the adhesive patch.[78,79]

Contraceptive ring

The contraceptive ring is a flexible, nonlatex plastic ring with a slow, continuous release of the hormonal components over the course of 3 weeks.[80] The ring is removed at the end of 3 weeks to allow for a withdrawal bleed for 3 to 7 days. Adolescents are more likely to report perfect use with the contraceptive vaginal ring, and it is often cited as being preferable to the patch or COC.[81] Acceptability of the contraceptive vaginal ring in adolescents was associated with positive feelings about genitals, knowledge of female anatomy, and comfort using a vaginal product.[82,83] When compared with COCs, adolescents report increased acceptability because of ease of use, and reported that they would recommend the method to their friends.[84]

Barrier Methods

Barrier methods are the only contraceptive methods that prevent STIs in addition to preventing pregnancy. Condom use at first intercourse increased from 48% in 1982 to 78% in 2006 to 2010, which is postulated to be a response to the HIV/AIDS epidemic.[6] Typical use of male condoms for contraception results in a failure rate of 18%.[24] Condom use requires the ability to communicate and negotiate with a partner, admit to risk of STI acquisition, and initiate use at the time of coitus, which can be challenging for adolescents.[85] Male partners exert a strong influence over adolescent women with regard to decision making about condom use.[86]

The increased use of LARC methods has resulted in a shift in the focus of condom use to highlight its role in STI prevention.[87] The rate of dual use among adolescents is 22.8%, and is lowest among LARC users.[88] The initiation of hormonal contraception is associated with a decrease in condom use in women of all ages.[89,90] Various behavioral intervention trials have been conducted to attempt to improve the rates of dual use, but have demonstrated little success.[91]

An important factor associated with increased dual use is the recommendation for consistent condom use by a health care provider at initiation of the hormonal contraceptive method.[92] Educating adolescents on the importance of condom use for STI prevention, the higher failure rate when compared with hormonal methods, and the importance of dual use for prevention of both pregnancy and STIs is critical to contraceptive counseling in adolescents.

REPRODUCTIVE HEALTH EDUCATION

Most adolescents have inadequate knowledge about contraceptive options, efficacy of methods, and unintended pregnancy.[93] Evidence-based reproductive health education programs are effective at reducing the rates of adolescent pregnancy and STIs, but are not widely implemented. Most reproductive health education curricula are taught during high school, and 46% of adolescent males and 33% of adolescent females report receiving no sexual health education before first intercourse.[94] Ninety-six percent of adolescents report receiving some form of sexual health education before leaving high school,[95] but only 70% of female adolescents report receiving instruction on contraception during their school curriculum.[95]

Adolescents report their most common sources of health education as their parents and peers, who often provide them with incorrect information, and Internet resources, many of which contain incorrect or incomplete information.[96,97] Adolescents who are already sexually active or who have received comprehensive sexual health education are more likely to access sexual health and contraceptive services.[98]

ACCESS TO CONTRACEPTION FOR ADOLESCENTS

Thirty-six percent of adolescents accessed contraceptive services from 2006 to 2010.[99] Nineteen percent accessed services in publicly funded clinics and 14% accessed services in private clinics.[99] The cost of contraceptive methods and parental knowledge of contraceptive use may deter adolescents from seeking effective contraception.[100]

State Laws and Consent

In 26 states and the District of Columbia, adolescents are able to consent to all contraceptive services regardless of circumstances.[101] Twenty states explicitly allow minors to consent for their own care only in certain circumstances, such as pregnancy, mental health services, testing for STIs, or contraception.[101] Knowledge of the specific state laws that affect adolescent reproductive health care and consent is an important asset for health care providers who care for adolescent patients.

Insurance

The Affordable Care Act (ACA) contraceptive mandate requires health insurance plans to provide coverage for all FDA-approved forms of contraception.[102] Adolescents who have insurance coverage under their parents' insurance plans may not want to use their insurance benefits for their contraception, and in these cases it may be acceptable to refer to publicly funded sources for further care.[100]

School-Based Health Centers

School-based health centers can be an important source of reproductive health education, STI testing, and contraception for adolescents. School-based health centers offer a variety of health care services for insured, underinsured, and uninsured school-aged children, and are funded by a combination of federal and private programs.[103] Eighty-five percent of school-based health centers offer reproductive health services, but only 37% provide any contraceptive services.[103,104] Restrictions on reproductive health services most commonly arise from school district policy but also from state and funding agency policies.[104]

Medicaid and Title X

The Department of Health and Human Services provides confidential federally funded family planning services (with the exception of abortion) through Medicaid and the Title

X program. One in 5 women who receives care at a Title X clinic is younger than 19 years.[105] State legislatures have attempted to restrict access by adolescents by attempting to pass legislation requiring parental consent for Title X family planning services,[106] but these efforts have been unsuccessful.

Examples of Successful Programs for Adolescents

Multiple programs have demonstrated increased use of more effective contraceptive methods and lower unintended pregnancy rates when the barriers of cost and access are removed. The Contraceptive CHOICE Project, conducted in St Louis, provided contraceptive counseling and initiation of a new method to 9256 women at no cost.[107] When evidence-based counseling was provided and the cost barrier was removed, 72% of the 1404 adolescents enrolled in the program chose a LARC method.[108] The pregnancy rate among teenagers enrolled in the CHOICE project was 34 per 1000 and the abortion rate was 9.7 per 1000, well below the national averages at the time of the study of 158.5 per 1000 and 41.5 per 1000 teenagers, respectively.[107]

The Colorado Family Planning Initiative, a privately funded reproductive health initiative, provided LARC methods at no cost to adolescents and young adults. Over the 4 years that the program was in place, the teenage birth rate and abortion rate for the state of Colorado were reduced by 29% and 34% respectively.[109]

SUMMARY

Despite the recent decrease in adolescent pregnancy rates, unintended pregnancy remains a significant problem in the United States.[8] The percentage of teens who engage in sexual intercourse increases dramatically over the course of adolescence, and adolescents face unique challenges when accessing contraception.[6]

Reproductive health visits beginning in early adolescence allow for development of a trusting provider-patient relationship, and permits early counseling on various risks and behaviors that adolescents may encounter.[13] LARC methods are recommended as first-line methods of contraception for adolescents because of their high efficacy, high continuation rates, and ease of use.[18] Counseling on anticipated side effects may play a role in decreasing the rates of discontinuation of contraceptive methods.[20] The use of condoms should always be encouraged for the prevention of STIs, and dual use should be emphasized at the time of contraceptive initiation.[92]

Reproductive health education curricula must be expanded to meet the educational needs of adolescents. The ACA contraceptive mandate and federal and private programs such as Title X, school-based health centers, and various private initiatives are helping to improve access to contraception for adolescents.

REFERENCES

1. Kost K, Henshaw S. U.S. Teenage pregnancies, births and abortions, 2010: national and state trends and trends by age, race and ethnicity. Guttmacher Institute; 2014. Available at: https://www.guttmacher.org/pubs/USTPtrends10.pdf.
2. Mosher WD, Jones J, Abma JC. Intended and unintended births in the United States: 1982-2010. Natl Health Stat Report 2012;(55):1–28.
3. Sedgh G, Finer LB, Bankole A, et al. Adolescent pregnancy, birth, and abortion rates across countries: levels and recent trends. J Adolesc Health 2015;56(2): 223–30.
4. The National Campaign to Prevent Teen and Unplanned Pregnancy. *Counting It Up*: Key Data. 2013. Available at: https://thenationalcampaign.org/resource/counting-it-key-data-2013.

5. Bridgeland JM, Dilulio JJ, Morison KB. Civic Enterprises. The silent epidemic: perspectives of high school dropouts. Bill and Melinda Gates Foundation; 2006.
6. Finer LB, Philbin JM. Sexual initiation, contraceptive use, and pregnancy among young adolescents. Pediatrics 2013;131(5):886–91.
7. Martinez G, Copen CE, Abma JC. Teenagers in the United States: sexual activity, contraceptive use, and childbearing, 2006-2010 National Survey of Family Growth. Vital Health Stat 23 2011;(31):1–35.
8. Guttmacher Institute. Unintended pregnancy in the United States fact sheet. Guttmacher Institute; 2015. Available at: http://www.guttmacher.org/pubs/FB-Unintended-Pregnancy-US.pdf.
9. Finer LB, Zolna MR. Shifts in intended and unintended pregnancies in the United States, 2001-2008. Am J Public Health 2014;104(Suppl 1):S43–8.
10. Finer LB, Jerman J, Kavanaugh ML. Changes in use of long-acting contraceptive methods in the United States, 2007-2009. Fertil Steril 2012;98(4):893–7.
11. Weinberger D, Elvevag B, Giedd J. The adolescent brain: a work in progress. Washington, DC: The National Campaign to Prevent Teen and Unplanned Pregnancy; 2005.
12. Kann L, Kinchen S, Shanklin SL, et al. Youth risk behavior surveillance—United States, 2013. MMWR Surveill Summ 2014;63(Suppl 4):1–168.
13. Committee on Adolescent Health Care. ACOG Committee Opinion no. 598: The initial reproductive health visit. Obstet Gynecol 2014;123(5):1143–7.
14. Ford C, English A, Sigman G. Confidential Health Care for Adolescents: position paper for the society for adolescent medicine. J Adolesc Health 2004;35(2):160–7.
15. Weinstock H, Berman S, Cates W, et al. Sexually transmitted diseases among American youth: incidence and prevalence estimates, 2000. Perspect Sex Reprod Health 2004;36(1):6–10.
16. Workowski KA, Bolan GA. Sexually transmitted diseases treatment guidelines, 2015. MMWR Recomm Rep 2015;64(RR–03):1–137.
17. Committee on Adolescent Health Care, Committee on Gynecologic Practice. Committee Opinion No. 582: addressing health risks of noncoital sexual activity. Obstet Gynecol 2013;122(6):1378–82.
18. Committee on Adolescent Health Care Long-Acting Reversible Contraception Working Group, The American College of Obstetricians and Gynecologists. Committee opinion no. 539: adolescents and long-acting reversible contraception: implants and intrauterine devices. Obstet Gynecol 2012;120(4):983–8.
19. Clark LR, Barnes-Harper KT, Ginsburg KR, et al. Menstrual irregularity from hormonal contraception: a cause of reproductive health concerns in minority adolescent young women. Contraception 2006;74(3):214–9.
20. Halpern V, Lopez LM, Grimes DA, et al. Strategies to improve adherence and acceptability of hormonal methods of contraception. Cochrane Database Syst Rev 2013;(10):CD00431.
21. Friedman JO. Factors associated with contraceptive satisfaction in adolescent women using the IUD. J Pediatr Adolesc Gynecol 2015;28(1):38–42.
22. Committee on Adolescence. Contraception for adolescents. Pediatrics 2014; 134(4):e1244–56.
23. Romero L, Pazol K, Warner L, et al. Vital signs: trends in use of long-acting reversible contraception among teens aged 15-19 years seeking contraceptive services—United States, 2005-2013. MMWR Morb Mortal Wkly Rep 2015; 64(13):363–9.
24. Trussell J. Contraceptive failure in the United States. Contraception 2011;83(5): 397–404.

25. McNicholas C, Maddipati R, Zhao Q, et al. Use of the etonogestrel implant and levonorgestrel intrauterine device beyond the U.S. Food and Drug Administration-approved duration. Obstet Gynecol 2015;125(3):599–604.
26. Mansour D, Korver T, Marintcheva-Petrova M, et al. The effects of Implanon on menstrual bleeding patterns. Eur J Contracept Reprod Health Care 2008; 13(Suppl 1):13–28.
27. Deokar AM, Jackson W, Omar HA. Menstrual bleeding patterns in adolescents using etonogestrel (ENG) implant. Int J Adolesc Med Health 2011;23(1):75–7.
28. Mansour D, Bahamondes L, Critchley H, et al. The management of unacceptable bleeding patterns in etonogestrel-releasing contraceptive implant users. Contraception 2011;83(3):202–10.
29. Wu JP, Pickle S. Extended use of the intrauterine device: a literature review and recommendations for clinical practice. Contraception 2014;89(6):495–503.
30. Gemzell-Danielsson K, Schellschmidt I, Apter D. A randomized, phase II study describing the efficacy, bleeding profile, and safety of two low-dose levonorgestrel-releasing intrauterine contraceptive systems and Mirena. Fertil Steril 2012; 97(3):616–22.e1-3.
31. Sivin I, Stern J, Diaz J, et al. Two years of intrauterine contraception with levonorgestrel and with copper: a randomized comparison of the TCu 380A and levonorgestrel 20 mcg/day devices. Contraception 1987;35(3):245–55.
32. Sanghera S, Roberts TE, Barton P, et al. Levonorgestrel-releasing intrauterine system vs. usual medical treatment for menorrhagia: an economic evaluation alongside a randomised controlled trial. PLoS One 2014;9(3):e91891.
33. Paterson H, Ashton J, Harrison-Woolrych M. A nationwide cohort study of the use of the levonorgestrel intrauterine device in New Zealand adolescents. Contraception 2009;79(6):433–8.
34. Stalnaker M, Esquivel P. Managing menorrhagia in a familial case of factor V deficiency. J Pediatr Adolesc Gynecol 2015;28(1):e9–12.
35. Rosenberg MJ, Foldesy R, Mishell DR Jr, et al. Performance of the TCu380A and Cu-Fix IUDs in an international randomized trial. Contraception 1996;53(4): 197–203.
36. Rivera R, Yacobson I, Grimes D. The mechanism of action of hormonal contraceptives and intrauterine contraceptive devices. Am J Obstet Gynecol 1999; 181(5 Pt 1):1263–9.
37. Ortiz ME, Croxatto HB. Copper-T intrauterine device and levonorgestrel intrauterine system: biological bases of their mechanism of action. Contraception 2007;75(6 Suppl):S16–30.
38. Centers for Disease Control and Prevention (CDC). U S. medical eligibility criteria for contraceptive use, 2010. MMWR Recomm Rep 2010;59(RR–4):1–86.
39. Milsom I, Andersson K, Jonasson K, et al. The influence of the Gyne-T 380S IUD on menstrual blood loss and iron status. Contraception 1995;52(3):175–9.
40. Grunloh DS, Casner T, Secura GM, et al. Characteristics associated with discontinuation of long-acting reversible contraception within the first 6 months of use. Obstet Gynecol 2013;122(6):1214–21.
41. Schmidt EO, James A, Curran KM, et al. Adolescent experiences with intrauterine devices: a qualitative study. J Adolesc Health 2015. [Epub ahead of print].
42. Turok DK, Godfrey EM, Wojdyla D, et al. Copper T380 intrauterine device for emergency contraception: highly effective at any time in the menstrual cycle. Hum Reprod 2013;28(10):2672–6.
43. Zhou L, Xiao B. Emergency contraception with Multiload Cu-375 SL IUD: a multicenter clinical trial. Contraception 2001;64(2):107–12.

44. Madden T, McNicholas C, Zhao Q, et al. Association of age and parity with intrauterine device expulsion. Obstet Gynecol 2014;124(4):718–26.
45. Deans EI, Grimes DA. Intrauterine devices for adolescents: a systematic review. Contraception 2009;79:418–23.
46. Chi I, Feldblum PJ, Rogers SM. IUD-related uterine perforation: an epidemiologic analysis of a rare event using an international dataset. Contracept Deliv Syst 1984;5:123–30.
47. Brown WM, Trouton K. Intrauterine device insertions: which variables matter? J Fam Plann Reprod Health Care 2014;40(2):117–21.
48. Hubacher D, Reyes V, Lillo S, et al. Pain from copper intrauterine device insertion: randomized trial of prophylactic ibuprofen. Am J Obstet Gynecol 2006; 195(5):1272–7.
49. Bednarek PH, Creinin MD, Reeves MF, et al. Prophylactic ibuprofen does not improve pain with IUD insertion: a randomized trial. Contraception 2015;91(3): 193–7.
50. Mody SK, Kiley J, Rademaker A, et al. Pain control for intrauterine device insertion: a randomized trial of 1% lidocaine paracervical block. Contraception 2012; 86(6):704–9.
51. Pergialiotis V, Vlachos DG, Protopappas A, et al. Analgesic options for placement of an intrauterine contraceptive: a meta-analysis. Eur J Contracept Reprod Health Care 2014;19(3):149–60.
52. Allen RH, Bartz D, Grimes DA, et al. Interventions for pain with intrauterine device insertion. Cochrane Database Syst Rev 2009;(3):CD007373.
53. Espey E, Singh RH, Leeman L, et al. Misoprostol for intrauterine device insertion in nulliparous women: a randomized controlled trial. Am J Obstet Gynecol 2014; 210(3):208.e1–5.
54. Division of Reproductive Health, National Center for Chronic Disease Prevention and Health Promotion, Centers for Disease Control and Prevention (CDC). U.S. Selected Practice Recommendations for Contraceptive Use, 2013: adapted from the World Health Organization selected practice recommendations for contraceptive use, 2nd edition. MMWR Recomm Rep 2013;62(RR–05):1–60.
55. Faúndes A, Telles E, Cristofoletti ML, et al. The risk of inadvertent intrauterine device insertion in women carriers of endocervical *Chlamydia trachomatis*. Contraception 1998;58(2):105–9.
56. American College of Obstetricians and Gynecologists. ACOG Practice Bulletin No. 121: long-acting reversible contraception: implants and intrauterine devices. Obstet Gynecol 2011;118(1):184–96.
57. Mohllajee AP, Curtis KM, Peterson HB. Does insertion and use of an intrauterine device increase the risk of pelvic inflammatory disease among women with sexually transmitted infection? A systematic review. Contraception 2006;73(2): 145–53.
58. Okusanya BO, Oduwole O, Effa EE. Immediate postabortal insertion of intrauterine devices. Cochrane Database Syst Rev 2014;(7):CD001777.
59. Steenland MW, Tepper NK, Curtis KM, et al. Intrauterine contraceptive insertion postabortion: a systematic review. Contraception 2011;84(5):447–64.
60. Ott MA, Sucato GS. Committee on Adolescence. Contraception for adolescents. Pediatrics 2014;134(4):e1257–81.
61. Polaneczky M, Liblanc M. Long-term depot medroxyprogesterone acetate (Depo-Provera) use in inner-city adolescents. J Adolesc Health 1998;23(2):81–8.
62. Jain J, Jakimiuk AJ, Bode FR, et al. Contraceptive efficacy and safety of DMPA-SC. Contraception 2004;70(4):269–75.

63. Zibners A, Cromer BA, Hayes J. Comparison of continuation rates for hormonal contraception among adolescents. J Pediatr Adolesc Gynecol 1999;12(2):90–4.
64. Bonny AE, Ziegler J, Harvey R, et al. Weight gain in obese and nonobese adolescent girls initiating depot medroxyprogesterone, oral contraceptive pills, or no hormonal contraceptive method. Arch Pediatr Adolesc Med 2006;160(1): 40–5.
65. Mangan SA, Larsen PG, Hudson S. Overweight teens at increased risk for weight gain while using depot medroxyprogesterone acetate. J Pediatr Adolesc Gynecol 2002;15(2):79–82.
66. Committee on Adolescent Healthcare, Committee on Gynecologic Practice. Committee opinion No. 602: depot medroxyprogesterone acetate and bone effects. Obstet Gynecol 2014;123(6):1398–402.
67. Cromer BA, Scholes D, Berenson A, et al. Depot medroxyprogesterone acetate and bone mineral density in adolescents—the black box warning: a position paper of the Society for Adolescent Medicine. J Adolesc Health 2006;39(2): 296–301.
68. Hall KS, Trussell J, Schwarz EB. Progestin-only contraceptive pill use among women in the United States. Contraception 2012;86(6):653–8.
69. American College of Obstetricians and Gynecologists. ACOG Practice Bulletin No. 110: noncontraceptive uses of hormonal contraceptives. Obstet Gynecol 2010;115(1):206–18.
70. Bitzer J, Simon JA. Current issues and available options in combined hormonal contraception. Contraception 2011;84(4):342–56.
71. van Hooff MH, Hirasing RA, Kaptein MB, et al. The use of oral contraceptives by adolescents for contraception, menstrual cycle problems or acne. Acta Obstet Gynecol Scand 1998;77(9):898–904.
72. Gallo MF, Lopez LM, Grimes DA, et al. Combination contraceptives: effects on weight. Cochrane Database Syst Rev 2014;(1):CD00398.
73. Committee on Gynecologic Practice. Committee Opinion Number 540: Risk of venous thromboembolism among users of drospirenone-containing oral contraceptive pills. Obstet Gynecol 2012;120(5):1239–42.
74. Lidegaard O, Nielsen LH, Skovlund CW, et al. Venous thrombosis in users of non-oral hormonal contraception: follow-up study, Denmark 2001-10. BMJ 2012;344:e2990.
75. Molloy GJ, Graham H, McGuinness H. Adherence to the oral contraceptive pill: a cross-sectional survey of modifiable behavioural determinants. BMC Public Health 2012;12:838.
76. Peipert JF, Zhao Q, Allsworth JE, et al. Continuation and satisfaction of reversible contraception. Obstet Gynecol 2011;117(5):1105–13.
77. Serfaty D. Medical aspects of oral contraceptive discontinuation. Adv Contracept 1992;8(Suppl 1):21–33.
78. Sucato GS, Land SR, Murray PJ, et al. Adolescents' experiences using the contraceptive patch versus pills. J Pediatr Adolesc Gynecol 2011;24(4):197–203.
79. Logsdon S, Richards J, Omar HA. Long-term evaluation of the use of the transdermal contraceptive patch in adolescents. ScientificWorldJournal 2004;4: 512–6.
80. Shimoni N, Westhoff C. Review of the vaginal contraceptive ring (NuvaRing). J Fam Plann Reprod Health Care 2008;34(4):247–50.
81. Gilliam ML, Neustadt A, Kozloski M, et al. Adherence an acceptability of the contraceptive ring compared with the pill among students: a randomized controlled trial. Obstet Gynecol 2010;115(3):503–10.

82. Carey AS, Chiappetta L, Tremont K, et al. The contraceptive vaginal ring: female adolescents' knowledge, attitudes and plans for use. Contraception 2007;76(6): 444–50.

83. Terrell LR, Tanner AE, Hensel DJ, et al. Acceptability of the vaginal contraceptive ring among adolescent women. J Pediatr Adolesc Gynecol 2011;24(4):204–10.

84. Stewart FH, Brown BA, Raine TR, et al. Adolescent and young women's experience with the vaginal ring and oral contraceptive pills. J Pediatr Adolesc Gynecol 2007;20(6):345–51.

85. Williams RL, Fortenberry JD. Update on adolescent condom use. Curr Opin Obstet Gynecol 2011;23(5):350–4.

86. Vasilenko SA, Kreager DA, Lefkowitz ES. Gender, contraceptive attitudes, and condom use in adolescent romantic relationships: a dyadic approach. J Res Adolesc 2015;25(1):51–62.

87. Williams RL, Fortenberry JD. Dual use of long-acting reversible contraceptives and condoms among adolescents. J Adolesc Health 2013;52(4 Suppl):S29–34.

88. Eisenberg DL, Allsworth JE, Zhao Q, et al. Correlates of dual-method contraceptive use: an analysis of the National Survey of Family Growth (2006-2008). Infect Dis Obstet Gynecol 2012;2012:717163.

89. Cushman LF, Romero D, Kalmuss D, et al. Condom use among women choosing long-term hormonal contraception. Fam Plann Perspect 1998;30(5):240–3.

90. Goldstein RL, Upadhyay UD, Raine TR. With pills, patches, rings, and shots: who still uses condoms? A longitudinal cohort study. J Adolesc Health 2013; 52(1):77–8.

91. Lopez LM, Stockton LL, Chen M, et al. Behavioral interventions for improving dual-method contraceptive use. Cochrane Database Syst Rev 2014;(3):CD010915.

92. Morroni C, Heartwell S, Edwards S, et al. The impact of oral contraceptive initiation on young women's condom use in 3 American cities: missed opportunities for intervention. PLoS One 2014;9(7):e101804.

93. Frost JJ, Lindberg LD, Finer LB. Young adults' contraceptive knowledge, norms and attitudes: associations with risk of unintended pregnancy. Perspect Sex Reprod Health 2012;44(2):107–16.

94. Facts on American teens' sources of information about sex fact sheet. Guttmacher Institute; 2012.

95. Martinez G, Abma J, Copen C. Educating teenagers about sex in the United States. NCHS Data Brief 2010;44:1–8.

96. Donaldson AA, Lindberg LD, Ellen JM, et al. Receipt of sexual health information from parents, teachers, and healthcare providers by sexually experienced U.S. adolescents. J Adolesc Health 2013;53(2):235–40.

97. Buhi ER, Daley EM, Oberne A, et al. Quality and accuracy of sexual health information web sites visited by young people. J Adolesc Health 2010;47(2):206–8.

98. Parkes A, Wight D, Henderson M. Teenagers' use of sexual health services: perceived need, knowledge and ability to access. J Fam Plann Reprod Health Care 2004;30(4):217–24.

99. Frost J. U.S. women's use of sexual and reproductive health services: trends, sources of care, and factors associated with use, 1995-2010. Guttmacher Institute; 2013. Available at: https://www.guttmacher.org/pubs/sources-of-care-2013.pdf.

100. American College of Obstetricians and Gynecologists Committee on Adolescent Healthcare. Guidelines for adolescent healthcare. 2nd edition. American College of Obstetricians and Gynecologists; 2011.

101. Guttmacher Institute. State policies in brief: an overview of minors' consent law. Guttmacher Institute; 2015. Available at: http://www.guttmacher.org/statecenter/ spibs/spib_OMCL.pdf.
102. Committee on Health Care for Underserved Women. Committee opinion no. 615: access to contraception. Obstet Gynecol 2015;125(1):250–5.
103. Boonstra HD. Meeting the sexual and reproductive health needs of adolescents in school-based health centers. Guttmacher Policy Review 2015;18(1). Available at: https://www.guttmacher.org/pubs/gpr/18/1/gpr1802115.pdf.
104. Fothergill K, Feijoo A. Family planning services at school-based health centers: findings from a national survey. J Adolesc Health 2000;27(3):166–9.
105. Fowler CI, Lloyd S, Gable J, et al. Family planning annual report: 2011 national summary. Research Triangle Park (NC): RTI International; 2012.
106. Adolescents' access to reproductive health services and information. Center for Reproductive Rights. September 3, 2010. Available at: http://www.reproductive rights.org/project/adolescents-access-to-reproductive-health-services-and-information. Accessed July 12, 2015.
107. Secura GM, Madden T, McNicholas C, et al. Provision of no-cost, long-acting contraception and teenage pregnancy. N Engl J Med 2014;371(14):1316–23.
108. Mestad R, Secura G, Allsworth JE, et al. Acceptance of long-acting reversible contraceptive methods by adolescent participants in the Contraceptive CHOICE Project. Contraception 2011;84(5):493–8.
109. Ricketts S, Klingler G, Schwalberg R. Game change in Colorado: widespread use of long-acting reversible contraceptives and rapid decline in births among young, low-income women. Perspect Sex Reprod Health 2014;46(3):125–32.

Safety and Efficacy of Contraceptive Methods for Obese and Overweight Women

Pamela S. Lotke, MD, MPH[a],*, Bliss Kaneshiro, MD, MPH[b]

KEYWORDS

- Obesity • Overweight • Contraception • Body mass index
- Hormonal contraception • Contraceptive efficacy

KEY POINTS

- Obesity is a public health challenge; many reproductive-age women are overweight or obese.
- Differences in pharmacokinetics and pharmacodynamics between normal weight and obese women using hormonal contraceptives have been noted, although efficacy does not appear to be severely impacted.
- Both obesity and estrogen-containing hormonal contraception increase the risk of venous thromboembolism (VTE). However, the absolute risk of VTE in obese, reproductive-age women using estrogen-containing contraceptives remains acceptably low.
- Studies suggest depo medroxyprogesterone is associated with more weight gain than other forms of hormonal contraception. Irrespective of contraceptive use, many women gain weight over time and retain weight gained during pregnancy.

INTRODUCTION

The obesity epidemic has become one of the greatest challenges to public health in the 21st century. More than one-third of adults in the United States are obese, resulting in 150 billion dollars in added medical costs each year.[1] Among women of reproductive age, 58.5% are overweight or obese.[2] Obese women who become pregnant have increased rates of gestational diabetes, hypertensive disease, macrosomia, and cesarean delivery, making the provision of contraception to obese women who wish to prevent pregnancy imperative.[3]

Disclosures: Dr P.S. Lotke serves on an international advisory board for Bayer Healthcare and as a clinical trainer for Nexplanon (Merck).
[a] MedStar Washington Hospital Center, Department of Obstetrics and Gynecology, 110 Irving Street Northwest, Washington, DC 20010, USA; [b] University of Hawaii John A. Burns School of Medicine, 1319 Punahou Street, #824, Honolulu, HI 96826, USA
* Corresponding author.
E-mail address: pamela.lotke@medstar.net

Obstet Gynecol Clin N Am 42 (2015) 647–657
http://dx.doi.org/10.1016/j.ogc.2015.07.005

Providing contraception to women of different weights raises 3 issues. First, contraceptives follow a one size fits all approach, with identical dosing regardless of body weight. No evidence suggests that contraceptives are ineffective in obese women. However, concerns have been raised about differences in the pharmacokinetics and pharmacodynamics of hormonal contraceptives that may alter efficacy in women of different body mass indices (BMIs). Secondly, estrogen-containing methods increase the risk of venous thromboembolism (VTE), for which obesity is an independent risk factor. Discussion is ongoing as to whether the risk of VTE in obese women who use combined hormonal contraceptives exceeds an acceptable level. Finally, women frequently have questions about the effect of contraceptive methods on weight gain. Hormonal medications are known to affect appetite, which may be concerning to women who are already above an ideal body weight.

These issues should be contextualized. A method with decreased efficacy in an obese woman will work better than no method. The increased risk of VTE related to combined hormonal contraceptives is lower than the risk of VTE associated with pregnancy. Studies suggest depo medroxyprogesterone acetate (DMPA) may be associated with some weight gain, but this weight gain may be lower than the weight retention associated with pregnancy. By comparing relative risks, both providers and patients will feel more confident about their contraceptive choices.

DEFINING OVERWEIGHT AND OBESITY

BMI, calculated by the weight in kilograms divided by height in meters squared, is a crude but useful indicator of body fat. The US Centers for Disease Control and Prevention (CDC) and the World Health Organization (WHO) have defined BMI categories as indicated in **Table 1**.[4]

EPIDEMIOLOGY OF OBESITY AND UNINTENDED PREGNANCY IN WOMEN OF DIFFERENT BODY MASS INDEX GROUPS

Differences in rates of obesity fall along racial and socioeconomic lines and mirror disparate rates of unintended pregnancy. Nearly 70% of Hispanic women and 80% of non-Hispanic black women of reproductive age are overweight or obese, compared with 55% of non-Hispanic reproductive age white women.[2] Approximately 30% of non-Hispanic black women have a BMI of 35 or greater compared with 15% of women

Table 1		
Weight categories and prevalence of obesity in reproductive-aged women		
Category	**BMI (kg/m²)**	**Prevalence (%)[a]**
Underweight	Below 18.5	40.5
Normal weight	18.5–24.9	
Overweight	25.0–29.9	25.5
Grade 1 obesity	30.0–34.9	15.1
Grade 2 obesity	35.0–39.9	11.3
Grade 3 obesity	40.0 and above	7.6

[a] Prevalence in Women age 20–39 years, 1999 to 2008, in the United States.
Data from Physical status: the use and interpretation of anthropometry. Report of a WHO Expert Committee. World Health Organ Tech Rep Ser 1995;854:1–452; and Flegal KM, Carroll MD, Kit BK, et al. Prevalence of obesity and trends in the distribution of body mass index among US adults, 1999–2010. JAMA 2012;307(5):491–7.

overall.[2] Women from higher income brackets and those with a college degree are less likely to be obese than women in lower income brackets and those with fewer years of education.[1]

Unintended pregnancy is also highest among minority women and those with fewer years of education. Black women have an unintended pregnancy rate of 92 pregnancies per 1000 population, and Hispanic women have a rate of 79 pregnancies per 1000 population, more than double that of non-Hispanic white women (38 pregnancies per 1000 population).[5] Reproductive age women without a high school degree have an unintended pregnancy rate of 101 pregnancies per 1000 women, which declines sharply as years of education increase.[5]

CONTRACEPTIVE USE AND SEXUAL BEHAVIOR IN WOMEN OF DIFFERENT BODY MASS INDICES

Contraceptive use and sexual behavior are 2 important factors that affect a woman's risk of pregnancy. Weight can affect body image, which plays a role in sexual behavior. Increased sexual interest and activity have been noted in obese women who lose weight.[6,7] In adult women, few differences have been noted in sexual behavior in women of different BMI groups.[8] In adolescents, white adolescent girls who were obese were more likely to have multiple sex partners and sex without a condom.[9] This relationship was not noted among black adolescent girls.[9]

Differences noted in nonuse of contraceptives by BMI may be more strongly associated with sociodemographic differences than weight itself.[10] Among sexually active reproductive age women, grade 2 and grade 3 obese women had the highest percentage of contraceptive nonuse at 33%, compared with 28% in normal weight women, 25.3% of grade 1 obese women, and 28.0% of overweight women (P<.05). However, after adjusting for race, ethnicity, age, cohabitation status, and the desire to become pregnant, no difference in contraceptive nonuse was noted between groups.[10] Some studies have noted that as weight increases, reliance on oral contraceptive pills and injectables decrease and reliance on sterilization, intrauterine devices (IUDs), and implants increase.[11] Other studies have not noted differences in contraceptive method choice between BMI groups.[12]

CONTRACEPTIVE EFFICACY IN OVERWEIGHT AND OBESE WOMEN
Pharmacokinetics, Pharmacodynamics, and Efficacy

Obesity may alter both the pharmacokinetics and pharmacodynamics of hormonal contraceptives. This may result in altered circulating levels of synthetic hormones, altered endogenous hormones based on feedback mechanisms, and possible ovulation. Minimal levels have been established as those necessary to prevent ovulation, which is an important function of hormonal contraceptive methods. Although ovulation is a surrogate for contraceptive efficacy, detecting ovulation is not the same as failed efficacy. In addition to suppression of follicular development and ovulation, most hormonal contraceptives work by making cervical mucus impermeable to sperm, impairing tubal motility, and making the endometrium less suitable for implantation. Even if pharmacodynamics are altered in obese women such that ovulation occasionally occurs, other contraceptive effects could still prevent pregnancy.

Intrauterine devices
Both the copper and levonorgestrel (LNG) IUD are highly effective regardless of weight given that the mechanism of action of the IUD is largely local. A prospective cohort study with nearly 6000 women–years of IUD use (LNG20 [initial release of

20 µg/d] and copper) reported the overall failure rate was less than 1 pregnancy per 100 woman–years and did not vary by BMI.[13]

Data from the European Active Surveillance Study, which enrolled over 61,000 women, also showed high efficacy for both types of IUDs. A significant proportion of women in this cohort were overweight or obese; 30% of women had a BMI between 25 and 30 kg/m^2; 10% had a BMI 30 to 35 kg/m^2, and 5% had a BMI over 35 kg/m^2.[14] Although they did not report weight specific data, the overall Pearl Index was 0.06 for the LNG20 IUD and 0.52 for the copper IUD.[15]

Implant

The etonogestrel implant appears to be highly effective regardless of body weight, although some studies suggest pharmacokinetics may be altered in obese women. Obese women have a lower maximum concentration, which cumulatively results in a woman being exposed to approximately 40% less etonogestrel over 3 years of implant use.[16] Concentrations of etonogestrel do remain above the threshold needed for contraceptive efficacy regardless of weight. The time to reach maximum concentration is the same in obese and normal-weight women, suggesting the etonogestrel's onset of action is similar between groups.[16]

The Contraceptive CHOICE project, which provided free contraception to over 9000 women in the St. Louis, Missouri, area, included 1168 women who initiated an etonogestrel implant during the study period. Thirty-seven percent of these women were normal weight; 28% were overweight, and 35% obese. Only 1 unintended pregnancy occurred in the group of women who initiated the implant, in a woman with a BMI of 30.7 kg/m^2. The resulting failure rate was 0.0 pregnancies per 100 woman–years for normal-weight women and 0.23 pregnancies per 100 woman–years for obese women.[13]

Injectable progestins (depo medroxyprogesterone acetate)

In a South African study designed to evaluate levels of intramuscular DMPA (150 mg) in women at the end of the dosing interval (11–14 weeks after injection), investigators reported no difference in medroxyprogesterone acetate (MPA) levels based on weight or BMI. Almost half of the women (46%) in this study had a BMI greater than or equal to 25 kg/m^2. Only 1 woman out of 94 had a level of MPA low enough for ovulation to be a concern.[17]

Another study examined the pharmacokinetics of the lower-dose subcutaneous DMPA (104 mg) in 5 normal-weight women, f obese women (BMI 30–39.9 kg/m^2) and 5 morbidly obese women (BMI >40 kg/m^2). Ovulation, as evidenced by progesterone level, did not occur in any woman after the first week of use. All women had MPA levels above that necessary to suppress ovulation up to 14 weeks after the injection, although a nonsignificant trend toward lower levels at every time point was noted in morbidly obese women.[18]

In a large multinational study examining the efficacy of subcutaneous DMPA, no pregnancies were reported in over 18,000 cycles of exposure. Almost half of the participants in the United States were overweight (26.2%) or obese (17.5%), as well as 27% of European and Asian participants.[19]

Oral contraceptives

Edelman and colleagues[20] reported altered pharmacokinetics with combined oral contraceptive pills. Obese women had a longer half-life of levonorgestrel, a lower peak concentration, and a longer time to reach steady state than normal-weight women.[20] Westhoff and colleagues[21] found that obese women taking combined oral contraceptive pills had a lower area under the curve and a lower maximum ethinyl estradiol level compared with normal-weight women. Smaller differences were noted in levonorgestrel levels for these parameters. Ethinyl estradiol and levonorgestrel troughs, which are likely more important to suppression of ovulation than maximum levels, were similar between BMI groups.

Altered pharmacodynamics have also been noted. Edelman and colleagues[20] noted more obese women showed estradiol levels and progesterone levels consistent with ovulation, suggesting less hypothalamic-pituitary-ovarian axis suppression compared with normal-weight women. Westhoff and colleagues[21] observed follicular diameters were larger in obese women taking combined oral contraceptive pills compared with normal-weight women, but this finding was not statistically different. In another study, obese and normal-weight women had similar follicular development, endogenous estradiol levels, Hoogland scores, and bleeding patterns.[22]

Most of the early studies on oral contraceptive pill efficacy were limited to women who were within 130% of their ideal body weight, leaving less data on efficacy in obese women. In 2009, Dinger and colleagues[23] published data from a cohort study of more than 52,000 women in the United States, 23.1% of whom were obese. The hazard ratio for pregnancy among women using a combined oral contraceptive pill with a BMI greater than 35 kg/m^2 was 1.5 times that of women with a BMI less than 35 kg/m^2.[24]

Other studies have not found differences in the risk of pregnancy in oral contraceptive pill users of different body weights. A study of 2810 women who were randomized to different pill formulations found a weak association between contraceptive failure and BMI that was not statistically different.[25] A phase 3 trial of an extended 91-day oral contraceptive regimen found no discernable differences in the failure rate across weight and BMI categories.[26] Data from more than 1500 women living in the United States, half of whom were using an oral contraceptive pill and half of whom were using a contraceptive patch or ring, also found no difference in failure rate by BMI.[27]

Vaginal ring

A pharmacokinetic study of normal-weight and obese etonogestrel (15 μg ethinyl estradiol/120 μg etonogestrel) vaginal ring users noted obese women had lower concentrations of ethinyl estradiol compared with normal-weight women but similar concentrations of etonogestrel.[28] Based on follicular development and serum progesterone levels, neither obese nor normal-weight women showed evidence of ovulation.[28] Another study examined the pharmacokinetics during extended use of the etonogestrel vaginal ring. After 21 to 42 days of continuous use, normal-weight and obese women had similar levels of etonogestrel, although obese women had lower levels of ethinyl estradiol.[29] Follicular development was minimal in both normal-weight and obese patients.[29] The authors concluded that a single contraceptive ring could be used for 6 weeks in both normal-weight and obese women.

McNicholas and colleagues[27] explored combined hormonal contraceptive failure in overweight and obese women in a 2013 analysis of the Contraceptive CHOICE project. Approximately 40% of combined hormonal contraceptive users were using an etonogestrel vaginal ring, with the others using the contraceptive patch or a pill. No difference in efficacy was noted between the methods or by BMI.

Transdermal patch

In a study to assess pharmacokinetics and ovarian suppression with use of a gestodene transdermal patch (0.55 mg ethinyl estradiol/2.1 mg gestodene), investigators purposefully recruited obese women, resulting in two-thirds of the study population having a BMI of 30 kg/m^2 or greater.[30] Six out of 173 women ovulated in either of the 2 study cycles. Ovulation did not correlate with BMI, although obese women were more likely to exhibit follicles of greater than 13 mm. Serum levels of follicle-stimulating hormone, luteinizing hormone, estradiol, and progesterone were similar between obese and normal-weight women. Body weight did not have an effect on gestodene levels. Clearance of ethinyl estradiol increased with increasing weight, although the minimal effect was unlikely to be clinically relevant.[30]

Efficacy studies of the currently available contraceptive patch (35 μg ethinyl estradiol/150 μg norelgestromin) included women up to 135% of their ideal body weight. A pooled analysis of patch studies found failure was low and uniform across the study population members who weighed less than 90 kg.[31] However, 5 of the 15 pregnancies that occurred were noted in the 3% of women who weighed more than 90 kg (198 pounds), suggesting efficacy may be lower in this group.[31]

CONTRACEPTIVE RISKS RELATED TO OBESITY
Guidance from the Medical Eligibility Criteria

Both the CDC and WHO maintain guidelines for contraceptive use in women with coexisting medical conditions known as the Medical Eligibility Criteria (MEC). The MEC delineate a level of risk for each contraceptive method in relation to various medical conditions[32,33] (**Table 2**).

The CDC MEC and WHO MEC consider use of combined hormonal methods, including the pill, patch, and ring, to be a level 2 for women with a BMI of 30 kg/m^2 or greater.[32,33] The Royal College of Obstetricians and Gynaecologists United Kingdom MEC also consider combined hormonal methods to be a level 2 for women with a BMI between 30 and 34.9 kg/m^2, but consider combined hormonal methods to be a level 3 for women with a BMI of 35 kg/m^2 or greater.[34]

Risks for Venous Thromboembolism

Nonhormonal forms of contraception, such as the copper IUD, and progestin-only methods, such as pills, DMPA, implants, and the levonorgestrel IUD, do not significantly increase the risk of VTE.[35] Estrogen is prothrombotic, resulting in an increased risk of VTE with estrogen-containing methods such as the oral contraceptive pill, patch, and ring. Obesity is also an independent risk factor for VTE.

Case–control studies have produced different estimates of the relative risk of VTE in obese versus normal-weight oral contraceptive pill users. A study from the Netherlands reported a 10-fold increased risk of VTE in overweight and obese women taking combined oral contraceptive pills compared with normal-weight women not taking pills.[36] In another study, normal-weight women taking combined oral contraceptive pills had an odds ratio of 4.2, overweight pill users an odds ratio of 11.6, and

Table 2 Medical eligibility criteria	
Categories of Medical Eligibility Criteria	
1	No restriction (method can be used)
2	Advantages generally outweigh theoretic or proven risks
3	Theoretic or proven risks usually outweigh the advantages
4	Unacceptable health risk (method not to be used)

Data from US Medical Eligibility Criteria 2010, adapted from World Health Organization Medical Eligibility Criteria. 4th edition. 2010. Available at: http://www.cdc.gov/reproductivehealth/UnintendedPregnancy/USMEC.htm. Accessed May 5, 2015; and WHO Medical Eligibility Criteria for contraceptive use. 4th edition. 2010. p. 121.

obese pill users an odds ratio of 23.8, compared with normal-weight women not using oral contraceptive pills.[37] A study from Denmark found that both oral contraceptive pills and obesity increased risk of VTE, but that there was no interaction between the risk factors.[38] A study from the United States reported oral contraceptive pill users with a BMI less than 30 kg/m^2 had 3.3 times the risk compared with non-users of the same BMI, while oral contraceptive pill users with a BMI over 30 had an odds ratio of 6.0.[39]

Markedly different estimates of relative risk make it difficult to determine whether the absolute risk of VTE in obese women using oral contraceptive pills is above an acceptable level.[40] The overall risk of VTE in combined oral contraceptive pill users is low, at 39 cases per 100,000 woman–years of exposure.[41] Based on available data, Trussell and colleagues noted the risk of VTE in obese women who use oral contraceptive pills is similar to the risk of VTE in older women using a combined oral contraceptive pill or younger smokers using a combined oral contraceptive pill. The authors concluded use of combined hormonal contraceptives among women with a BMI above 35 kg/m^2 should not be restricted based on concerns for safety.

Use of any contraceptive method in obese women is safer than pregnancy. Rates of VTE during the antepartum period, third trimester, and first 6 weeks postpartum are 99, 182, and 468 cases per 100,000 woman–years, respectively.[42] The risk of VTE during pregnancy is even higher in obese women. One study from Denmark showed obese pregnant women with a BMI over 30 kg/m^2 had an odds ratio of 5.3 of developing VTE and an odds ratio of 14.9 for developing pulmonary embolism relative to normal-weight pregnant women.[43]

EFFECTS OF CONTRACEPTION ON WEIGHT

Weight gain is a frequently mentioned concern for women selecting a contraceptive method. Most methods of contraception, including combined oral contraceptive pills, are not associated with weight gain,[44,45] although weight gain is a commonly cited reason for method discontinuation.[46,47] IUDs, implants, vaginal rings, and the contraceptive patch are also not associated with weight gain.

DMPA has been associated with weight gain in some studies, although reports in the medical literature on this topic vary. A small, randomized controlled trial did not observe changes in food intake, metabolic expenditures, or weight gain in DMPA users compared with nonusers over a 3 month interval.[48] Observational studies have reported DMPA-associated weight gain varies by age, race, weight at initiation, and rate of weight gain. Adolescents who gain more than 5% of their body weight in the first 6 months of use tend to gain significantly more weight over time than those who gain less weight initially.[49] In a 3-year observational study, normal-weight women gained more weight (4.5 kg) than overweight (3.4 kg) or obese women (1.9 kg). Women who were not using DMPA also gained weight over the study period (1.2 kg in normal-weight women).[50] Data from the Contraceptive CHOICE project noted 12-month weight gain was higher in women using the implant (2.1 kg) and DMPA (2.2 kg) than the levonorgestrel IUD (1.0 kg) and copper IUD (0.2 kg).[45] However, after adjusting for differences in age and race, no difference in weight gain was seen in implant, DMPA, and levonorgestrel IUD users compared with copper IUD users.

Women of all weights will have a negative perception of a contraceptive method that hampers weight loss or contributes to weight gain. Importantly, most women will gain weight as they progress through their reproductive years. In a study of 1700 Brazilian women using a copper IUD, weight gain over time was noted; weight increased by 2.7 kg after 5 years and 4.0 kg after 7 years.[51] Contraceptives prevent pregnancy, a condition that is associated with weight gain. In a study done in the United States with 2510 women, 40% of whom were normal weight at the start of pregnancy, three-quarters were heavier than their prepregnancy weight at 1-year postpartum. Nearly half (47.4%) were more than 10 pounds heavier, and almost one-quarter (24%) were more than 20 pounds heavier.[52] When considering contraceptive options, weight gain from pregnancy and weight gain accumulated over time should be considered.

SUMMARY

Although obesity alters the pharmacokinetics and pharmacodynamics of hormonal contraceptives, efficacy does not appear to be significantly impacted. Obesity increases a woman's risk for VTE, as does the use of estrogen-containing contraception. However, the combined risk remains acceptably low, and all methods should be considered safe in obese women who do not have other coexisting medical conditions. Use of combined hormonal contraceptives, progestin implants, and the IUD are not associated with weight gain. Certain groups appear to be susceptible to weight gain with DMPA including those who demonstrate higher weight gain with initiation of the method. The risk of weight gain and VTE is higher with pregnancy than with use of any contraceptive method. Consequently, the most important factor is choosing a method is whether a woman will be satisfied and compliant with the method.

Health care providers will care for women of all body weights on a daily basis. In order to provide effective guidance, clinicians should understand the safety and efficacy of contraceptive methods in relation to weight. Given the increased health risks of unintended pregnancy in obese women, the most effective methods, including the IUD and implant, should be prioritized.

REFERENCES

1. Coutinho E, Segal S. Is menstruation obsolete? New York: Oxford University Press; 1999.
2. Ogden CL, Carroll MD, Kit BK, et al. Prevalence of childhood and adult obesity in the United States, 2011-2012. JAMA 2014;311(8):806–14.
3. American College of Obstetricians and Gynecologists. Committee opinion no. 549: obesity in pregnancy. Obstet Gynecol 2013;121(1):213–7.
4. Physical status: the use and interpretation of anthropometry. Report of a WHO Expert Committee. World Health Organ Tech Rep Ser 1995;854:1–452.
5. Finer LB, Zolna MR. Shifts in intended and unintended pregnancies in the United States, 2001-2008. Am J Public Health 2014;104(Suppl 1):S43–8.
6. Hawke A, O'Brien P, Watts JM, et al. Psychosocial and physical activity changes after gastric restrictive procedures for morbid obesity. Aust N Z J Surg 1990; 60(10):755–8.
7. Werlinger K, King TK, Clark MM, et al. Perceived changes in sexual functioning and body image following weight loss in an obese female population: a pilot study. J Sex Marital Ther 1997;23(1):74–8.
8. Kaneshiro B, Jensen JT, Carlson NE, et al. Body mass index and sexual behavior. Obstet Gynecol 2008;112(3):586–92.
9. Leech TG, Dias JJ. Risky sexual behavior: a race-specific social consequence of obesity. J Youth Adolesc 2012;41(1):41–52.

10. Vahratian A, Barber JS, Lawrence JM, et al. Family-planning practices among women with diabetes and overweight and obese women in the 2002 National Survey For Family Growth. Diabetes Care 2009;32(6):1026–31.
11. Schraudenbach A, McFall S. Contraceptive use and contraception type in women by body mass index category. Womens Health Issues 2009;19(6):381–9.
12. Kaneshiro B, Edelman A, Carlson N, et al. The relationship between body mass index and unintended pregnancy: results from the 2002 National Survey of Family Growth. Contraception 2008;77(4):234–8.
13. Xu H, Wade JA, Peipert JF, et al. Contraceptive failure rates of etonogestrel subdermal implants in overweight and obese women. Obstet Gynecol 2012;120(1):21–6.
14. Heinemann K, Reed S, Moehner S, et al. Risk of uterine perforation with levonorgestrel-releasing and copper intrauterine devices in the European Active Surveillance Study on Intrauterine Devices. Contraception 2015;91(4):274–9.
15. Heinemann K, Reed S, Moehner S, et al. Comparative contraceptive effectiveness of levonorgestrel-releasing and copper intrauterine devices: the European Active Surveillance Study for Intrauterine Devices. Contraception 2015;91(4):280–3.
16. Mornar S, Chan L-N, Mistretta S, et al. Pharmacokinetics of the etonogestrel contraceptive implant in obese women. Am J Obstet Gynecol 2012;207(2):110.e1–6.
17. Smit J, Botha J, McFadyen L, et al. Serum medroxyprogesterone acetate levels in new and repeat users of depot medroxyprogesterone acetate at the end of the dosing interval. Contraception 2004;69(1):3–7.
18. Segall-Gutierrez P, Taylor D, Liu X, et al. Follicular development and ovulation in extremely obese women receiving depo-medroxyprogesterone acetate subcutaneously. Contraception 2010;81(6):487–95.
19. Jain J, Jakimiuk AJ, Bode FR, et al. Contraceptive efficacy and safety of DMPA-SC. Contraception 2004;70(4):269–75.
20. Edelman AB, Carlson NE, Cherala G, et al. Impact of obesity on oral contraceptive pharmacokinetics and hypothalamic–pituitary–ovarian activity. Contraception 2009;80(2):119–27.
21. Westhoff CL, Torgal AH, Mayeda ER, et al. Pharmacokinetics of a combined oral contraceptive in obese and normal-weight women. Contraception 2010;81(6):474–80.
22. Westhoff CL, Torgal AH, Mayeda ER, et al. Ovarian suppression in normal-weight and obese women during oral contraceptive use: a randomized controlled trial. Obstet Gynecol 2010;116(2 Part 1):275–83.
23. Dinger JC, Cronin M, Möhner S, et al. Oral contraceptive effectiveness according to body mass index, weight, age, and other factors. Am J Obstet Gynecol 2009;201(3):263.e1–9.
24. Dinger J, Minh TD, Buttmann N, et al. Effectiveness of oral contraceptive pills in a large U.S. cohort comparing progestogen and regimen. Obstet Gynecol 2011;117(1):33–40.
25. Burkman RT, Fisher AC, Wan GJ, et al. Association between efficacy and body weight or body mass index for two low-dose oral contraceptives. Contraception 2009;79(6):424–7.
26. Westhoff CL, Hait HI, Reape KZ. Body weight does not impact pregnancy rates during use of a low-dose extended-regimen 91-day oral contraceptive. Contraception 2012;85(3):235–9.
27. McNicholas C, Zhao Q, Secura G, et al. Contraceptive failures in overweight and obese combined hormonal contraceptive users. Obstet Gynecol 2013;121(3):585–92.

28. Westhoff CL, Torgal AH, Mayeda ER, et al. Pharmacokinetics and ovarian suppression during use of a contraceptive vaginal ring in normal-weight and obese women. Am J Obstet Gynecol 2012;207(1):39.e1–6.

29. Dragoman M, Petrie K, Torgal A, et al. Contraceptive vaginal ring effectiveness is maintained during 6 weeks of use: a prospective study of normal BMI and obese women. Contraception 2013;87(4):432–6.

30. Westhoff CL, Reinecke I, Bangerter K, et al. Impact of body mass index on suppression of follicular development and ovulation using a transdermal patch containing 0.55-mg ethinyl estradiol/2.1-mg gestodene: a multicenter, open-label, uncontrolled study over three treatment cycles. Contraception 2014; 90(3):272–9.

31. Zieman M, Guillebaud J, Weisberg E, et al. Contraceptive efficacy and cycle control with the Ortho Evra/Evra transdermal system: the analysis of pooled data. Fertil Steril 2002;77(2 Suppl 2):S13–8.

32. US Medical Eligibility Criteria 2010, adapted from World Health Organization Medical Eligibility Criteria. 4th edition. 2010. Available at: http://www.cdc.gov/reproductivehealth/UnintendedPregnancy/USMEC.htm. Accessed May 5, 2015.

33. World Health Organization. Medical eligibility criteria for contraceptive use: fourth edition. 2010. Available at: http://whqlibdoc.who.int/publications/2010/9789241563888_eng.pdf. Accessed May 5, 2015.

34. UK Medical eligibility criteria for contraceptive use. 2009. Available at: http://www.fsrh.org/pdfs/UKMEC2009.pdf. Accessed May 5, 2015.

35. Blanco-Molina MA, Lozano M, Cano A, et al. Progestin-only contraception and venous thromboembolism. Thromb Res 2012;129(5):e257–62.

36. Abdollahi M, Cushman M, Rosendaal FR. Obesity: risk of venous thrombosis and the interaction with coagulation factor levels and oral contraceptive use. Thromb Haemost 2003;89(3):493–8.

37. Pomp ER, Le Cessie S, Rosendaal FR, et al. Risk of venous thrombosis: obesity and its joint effect with oral contraceptive use and prothrombotic mutations. Br J Haematol 2007;139(2):289–96.

38. Lidegaard Ø, Edström B, Kreiner S. Oral contraceptives and venous thromboembolism: a five-year national case-control study. Contraception 2002;65(3):187–96.

39. Sidney S, Petitti DB, Soff GA, et al. Venous thromboembolic disease in users of low-estrogen combined estrogen–progestin oral contraceptives. Contraception 2004;70(1):3–10.

40. Trussell J, Guthrie KA, Schwarz EB. Much ado about little: obesity, combined hormonal contraceptive use and venous thrombosis. Contraception 2008;77(3): 143–6.

41. Nightingale AL, Lawrenson RA, Simpson EL, et al. The effects of age, body mass index, smoking and general health on the risk of venous thromboembolism in users of combined oral contraceptives. Eur J Contracept Reprod Health Care 2000;5(4):265–74.

42. Abdul Sultan A, Tata LJ, Grainge MJ, et al. The incidence of first venous thromboembolism in and around pregnancy using linked primary and secondary care data: a population based cohort study from England and comparative meta-analysis. PLoS One 2013;8(7):e70310.

43. Larsen TB, Sørensen HT, Gislum M, et al. Maternal smoking, obesity, and risk of venous thromboembolism during pregnancy and the puerperium: a population-based nested case–control study. Thromb Res 2007;120(4):505–9.

44. Gallo MF, Lopez LM, Grimes DA, et al. Combination contraceptives: effects on weight. Cochrane Database Syst Rev 2014;(1):CD003987.

45. Vickery Z, Madden T, Zhao Q, et al. Weight change at 12 months in users of three progestin-only contraceptive methods. Contraception 2013;88(4):503–8.
46. Rosenberg MJ, Waugh MS, Meehan TE. Use and misuse of oral contraceptives: risk indicators for poor pill taking and discontinuation. Contraception 1995;51(5): 283–8.
47. Funk S, Miller MM, Mishell DR Jr, et al. Safety and efficacy of Implanon™, a single-rod implantable contraceptive containing etonogestrel. Contraception 2005;71(5):319–26.
48. Pelkman CL, Chow M, Heinbach RA, et al. Short-term effects of a progestational contraceptive drug on food intake, resting energy expenditure, and body weight in young women. Am J Clin Nutr 2001;73(1):19–26.
49. Bonny AE, Secic M, Cromer B. Early weight gain related to later weight gain in adolescents on depot medroxyprogesterone acetate. Obstet Gynecol 2011; 117(4):793–7.
50. Pantoja M, Medeiros T, Baccarin MC, et al. Variations in body mass index of users of depot-medroxyprogesterone acetate as a contraceptive. Contraception 2010; 81(2):107–11.
51. Hassan DF, Petta CA, Aldrighi JM, et al. Weight variation in a cohort of women using copper IUD for contraception. Contraception 2003;68(1):27–30.
52. Endres LK, Straub H, McKinney C, et al. Postpartum weight retention risk factors and relationship to obesity at 1 year. Obstet Gynecol 2015;125(1):144–52.

Contraceptive Method Initiation

Using the Centers for Disease Control and Prevention Selected Practice Guidelines

Wan-Ju Wu, MD, MPH, Alison Edelman, MD, MPH*

KEYWORDS

- Contraception • Pregnancy • Screening tests • Pregnancy prevention
- CDC Selected Practice Guidelines

KEY POINTS

- A woman can start most contraceptive methods immediately if the provider is reasonably certain that she is not pregnant.
- Few tests or examinations are necessary to initiate a contraceptive method.
- No specific follow-up visits after initiation of contraception are required. If any subsequent follow-up visits occur, providers should address a woman's satisfaction with her method, concerns about use, and changes in health status that may affect eligibility for continued use of the method.

INTRODUCTION

Women have a variety of safe and effective methods available to prevent or delay pregnancy, but the number of options now available can make the provision of care complicated for providers. Clinical guidelines now exist to help providers deliver evidence-based contraceptive care. The US Medical Eligibility Criteria for Contraceptive Use (MEC) describe who can safely use a method based on a woman's preexisting medical conditions and circumstances.[1] The US Selected Practice Recommendations (SPR) is a companion document that focuses on how providers can use contraceptive methods most effectively as well as problem-solve common issues that may arise.[2] These guidelines have been created to help clinicians in the provision of care and to decrease barriers that prevent or delay a woman from obtaining a

Disclosures: The authors have nothing to disclose.
Department of Obstetrics and Gynecology, Oregon Health & Science University, 3181 Southwest Sam Jackson Park Road, Portland, OR 97239, USA
* Corresponding author.
E-mail address: edelmana@ohsu.edu

Obstet Gynecol Clin N Am 42 (2015) 659–667
http://dx.doi.org/10.1016/j.ogc.2015.07.006
0889-8545/15/$ – see front matter © 2015 Elsevier Inc. All rights reserved.

obgyn.theclinics.com

desired method that would place them at risk for pregnancy. This article summarizes the SPR on timing of contraceptive initiation, examinations, tests needed prior to starting a method, and any necessary follow-up.

METHOD INITIATION

Initiation of a contraceptive method requires a provider and woman to jointly weigh the risks and benefits of the potential choice. The main risk is typically around estrogen-containing methods (pills, patches, and rings). In most instances, the balance falls in favor of starting a method, because the risks of pregnancy typically outweigh the risks of using a contraceptive method. A thorough medical history can assist a provider in determining which methods of contraception a woman is eligible for. As discussed previously, the MEC should be used to aid a provider in deciding who can use a method. Certain medical conditions may place a particular method in MEC category 4, which indicates, "A condition that represents an unacceptable health risk if the contraceptive method is used."[3] The MEC does not take into account the risks of use compared with the risks of pregnancy.

Once possible contraindications or precautions to a method have been reviewed, most women can start contraception at any time as long as the provider is reasonably certain that she is not pregnant. The Centers for Disease Control and Prevention (CDC) recommends the following criteria for assessment of pregnancy (**Box 1**).

Although most clinical practices routinely perform urine pregnancy tests (UPTs), the CDC guidelines favor using a detailed history to determine risk of pregnancy and only using a UPT as an adjunct. Data show that this checklist of criteria has high negative predicative value but varies widely in terms of sensitivity and specificity.[4] If a woman does not meet criteria to be reasonably certain that she is not pregnant, then a negative pregnancy test does not provide additional reassurance regarding pregnancy status. UPTs have to be interpreted in the context of timing of the missed menses, unprotected intercourse, and recent pregnancy. UPTs are highly sensitive but only after implantation has occurred. Implantation occurs on the first day of the missed period in only 90% of pregnancies.[4] This means that as many as 10% of pregnancies can be missed if a UPT is performed on the first day of a woman's missed menses.[5] A UPT does not detect a pregnancy resulting from very recent intercourse. Furthermore,

---

Box 1
How to be reasonably certain that a woman is not pregnant

A health care provider can be reasonably certain that a woman is not pregnant if she has no symptoms or signs of pregnancy and meets any one of the following criteria:

- Is less than or equal to 7 days after the start of normal menses
- Has not had sexual intercourse since the start of last normal menses
- Has been correctly and consistently using a reliable method of contraception
- Is less than or equal to 7 days after spontaneous or induced abortion
- Is within 4 weeks postpartum
- Is fully or nearly fully breastfeeding (exclusively breastfeeding or the vast majority [≥85%] of feeds are breastfeeds), amenorrheic, and less than 6 months postpartum

Adapted from World Health Organization. Selected practice recommendations for contraceptive use. 2nd edition. Geneva: WHO; 2004. Available at: http://whqlibdoc.who.int/publications/2004/9241562846.pdf. Accessed May 5, 2015.

after a recent pregnancy (postpartum, abortion, or miscarriage), human chorionic gonadotropin remains detectable for several weeks, resulting in positive UPTs.[6,7]

As discussed previously, once a provider is reasonably certain that a woman is not pregnant and she has no contraindications to use, it is safe to initiate all methods of contraception at any time (**Table 1**). With the exception of the copper (Cu) intrauterine device (IUD), a back-up method may be needed, depending on where a woman is in the menstrual cycle when the contraceptive method is initiated. A back-up method

Table 1
When to start using specific contraceptive methods

Contraceptive Method	When to Start (if the Provider is Reasonably Certain that the Woman is Not Pregnant)	Additional Contraception (ie, Back-Up) Needed	Examinations or Tests Needed Before Initiation[a]
Cu-IUD	Anytime	Not needed	Bimanual examination and cervical inspection[b]
LNG-IUD	Anytime	If >7 d after menses started, use back-up method or abstain for 7 d	Bimanual examination and cervical inspection[b]
Implant	Anytime	If >5 d after menses started, use back-up method or abstain for 7 d	None
Injectable	Anytime	If >7 d after menses started, use back-up method or abstain for 7 d	None
CHC	Anytime	If >5 d after menses started, use back-up method or abstain for 7 d	Blood pressure measurement
Progestin-only pill	Anytime	If >5 d after menses started, use back-up method or abstain for 2 d	None

Abbreviation: U.S. MEC, *U.S. Medical Eligibility Criteria for Contraceptive Use, 2010.*

[a] Weight (BMI) measurement is not needed to determine medical eligibility for any methods of contraception because all methods can be used (U.S. MEC 1) or generally can be used (U.S. MEC 2) among obese women (see **Box 2**). Measuring weight and calculating BMI (weight [kg]/height [m^2]) at baseline might be helpful, however, for monitoring any changes and counseling women who might be concerned about weight change perceived associated with their contraceptive method.

[b] Most women do not require additional STD screening at the time of IUD insertion if they have already been screened according to CDC's *STD Treatment Guidelines* (available at: http://www.cdc.gov/std/treatment). If a woman has not been screened according to guidelines, screening can be performed at the time of IUD insertion, and insertion should not be delayed. Women with purulent cervicitis or current chlamydial infection or gonorrhea should not undergo IUD insertion (U.S. MEC 4). Women who have a very high individual likelihood of STD exposure (eg, those with a currently infected partner) generally should not undergo IUD insertion (U.S. MEC 3) (see **Table 1**). For these women, IUD insertion should be delayed until appropriate testing and treatment occurs.

From Division of Reproductive Health, National Center for Chronic Disease Prevention and Health Promotion, Centers for Disease Control and Prevention (CDC). U.S. Selected Practice Recommendations for Contraceptive Use. 2013.

should be used when starting an implant, combined hormonal contraceptive (CHC), and progestin-only pill if it has been greater than 5 days since a woman's last menstrual period (LMP). If initiating levonorgestrel-releasing IUD (LNG-IUD) or depot medroxyprogesterone acetate (DMPA), a back-up method is recommended if it has been greater than 7 days since LMP. When switching from one contraceptive method to another, a new method generally can be initiated immediately as along as the provider is reasonably certain that the woman is not pregnant. If the woman has stopped contraceptive use for a period of time, has not been using contraception correctly or continuously, has had recent unprotected intercourse, or has started her next menses, a back-up method may also be needed.[8]

Although it makes intuitive sense that starting contraception as soon as possible should decrease the risk of pregnancy for women, data have not consistently shown that the overall short-term or long-term method effectiveness is changed by timing of method initiation.[9] Specifically, for Cu-IUDs and LNG-IUDs, a systematic review did not suggest differences in continuation, expulsion, removal, or pregnancy rates when the devices are inserted at different times of the menstrual cycle.[10] Studies have examined the quick start method for CHCs, where a woman starts her contraceptive method either on the same day or shortly after her clinic visit, compared with the conventional start method, where the woman starts contraception with her next menses. The studies were not powered to detect a difference in effectiveness, but they did find improved continuation rates early in use, although this advantage diminished over time.[11] There were no differences in method adherence and bleeding patterns; however, 3 of the trials did demonstrate greater patient satisfaction with an immediate start.[12–14]

In instances where the provider cannot be reasonably certain that the woman is not pregnant, the benefits of starting contraception still generally outweigh the risks for all methods except for IUDs. Hormonal contraceptive methods do not have any known associated teratogenic or abortifacient effects.[15–17] If it has been less than 5 days since unprotected intercourse, it is reasonable to offer a woman emergency contraception and then have her start her method immediately after. A follow-up pregnancy test in 2 to 4 weeks should be performed.

In contrast, pregnancies with IUDs in place are at high risk for devastating complications including spontaneous abortion, septic abortion, preterm delivery, and chorioamnionitis.[18]

If pregnancy cannot be confidently ruled out, the SPR recommends that the provider offer an alternative short-term method, such as the pills, patch, ring, or DMPA, and delay placement until she can be certain that the woman is not pregnant. An exception is placement of a Cu-IUD within 5 days of unprotected intercourse because it can be used as an emergency contraceptive method and then continued as an ongoing form of contraception. Although adverse pregnancy outcomes are clearly associated with having an IUD in situ, the data also point to improved outcomes with immediate removal.[18] In practice, some providers counsel a woman on the risks and benefits and still place an IUD, ensuring that she will take a pregnancy test within the next 2 to 4 weeks, with immediate removal if the woman is found pregnant.

A woman's visit to initiate contraception can be an important time to promote continuation and correct usage of the method. Evidence shows that providing more pill packs at the time (12–13 packs vs 1 pack) of prescribing improves continuation rates as well as decreases rates of pregnancy tests and actual pregnancies.[19–21] Greater initial pill supply is also associated with lower costs to the health care system.[22] These initiation visits are also valuable opportunities for expanded counseling. Studies indicate that focused counseling on expected bleeding patterns and reassurance that the bleeding is benign reduce discontinuation rates for DMPA.[23,24] It is reasonable to assume that similar counseling on potential side effects when initiating other methods of contraception would have similar impact.

SPECIAL CIRCUMSTANCES

The SPR provides guidelines for initiating each contraceptive method under special circumstances, including when a woman is amenorrheic as well as in the postpregnancy (postpartum, abortion, or miscarriage) period. The principles for initiation of a contraceptive method are similar for women who have amenorrhea as those who have normal cycles. Any method can be initiated at any time if the provider is reasonably certain that the woman is not pregnant. The recommendations for use of a back-up method are also the same as for women who do not have amenorrhea.

Postpartum

During the postpartum period, many previously uninsured or underinsured women have access to health care and a heightened motivation to avoid another pregnancy. This can be the ideal time to initiate contraception. Decreasing short-interval pregnancies improves the health of mothers and infants. Many women wait until the 6-week postpartum visit to initiate contraception; however, ovulation in nonbreastfeeding women may occur as soon as 4 weeks postpartum. Studies from several different countries have shown that anywhere from 30% to 60% of women resume intercourse by the sixth week postpartum.[25] Although not specifically addressed in the SPR, providers should encourage women to initiate a contraceptive method by the third week postpartum.

For women who are breastfeeding, lactational amenorrhea method (LAM) is effective contraception only if a woman is less than 6 months postpartum, exclusively breastfeeding (>85% of the time), and has amenorrhea. Exclusively breastfeeding entails day and night feedings that are less than 4 to 6 hours apart; otherwise, a back-up contraceptive method is recommended. Pumping or expression of milk by hand is not as vigorous as suckling and may not suppress ovulation as effectively, potentially placing women at increased risk for ovulation and fertility.[26] Due to LAM's strict criteria, few women actually enjoy the full contraceptive advantages of breastfeeding.

The MEC provides guidelines for initiation of contraceptive methods in the postpartum period. CHCs are contraindicated in the first 3 weeks postpartum for all women because they can contribute to the already increased risk for venous thromboembolic events (VTEs). Women without additional risk factors for VTEs (eg, postcesarean section or other medical comorbidities) may initiate CHC at 3 weeks postpartum. For those women who do have additional risk factors for VTE, from 3 to 6 weeks postpartum the risks of CHC use generally outweigh the benefits and should not be used. In addition to the VTE risks, for breastfeeding women CHCs theoretically can have negative effects on milk production.[27] This is based on few data. A recent systematic review examined the impact of CHC versus nonhormonal contraceptive methods versus progestin-only contraceptive methods on lactation. The overall conclusion is that there is little evidence of negative effects with any particular method.[28]

All other contraceptive methods can be initiated at any time postpartum, including immediately postpartum in breastfeeding and nonbreastfeeding women if pregnancy has been reasonably ruled out. As long as there is no concern for intra-amniotic infections, IUDs can be inserted immediately postpartum without any associated increase in complication rates. Patients should be counseled on the higher expulsion rates when an IUD is inserted less than 28 days postpartum.[29,30]

Postabortion

All methods of contraception, including CHCs, can be initiated immediately postabortion.[31] Exceptions are women who have had a septic abortion, in which case IUDs should not be inserted.

EXAMINATIONS AND TESTS PRIOR TO INITIATION

With healthy young women, few tests are necessary prior to initiation of a contraceptive method. Women who have specific medical conditions may need additional workup prior to initiation. Providers need to address these women on an individual basis because this is not addressed by the SPR.

Intrauterine Device

A bimanual examination and a cervical examination are necessary prior to insertion of an IUD. If a woman has been screened per the CDC sexually transmitted disease (STD) testing guidelines, additional screening is not necessary at the time of insertion unless there is concern for new risk factors, that is, a current infected partner or clinical evidence of infection (**Box 2**). For these women, IUD insertion should be delayed until testing and treatment have been completed. Women can be placed on a short-term bridging method until the IUD can be placed. Women who have not undergone routine STD screening per the CDC guidelines should be screened if necessary at the time of insertion. There is no need to wait for the test results prior to insertion. Evidence indicates higher risk for pelvic inflammatory disease if a woman has an STD at the time of IUD insertion, but overall rates are low.[32]

Box 2
Centers for Disease Control and Prevention sexually transmitted disease and HIV screening guidelines

- All adults and adolescents from ages 13 to 64 should be tested at least once for HIV.

- Annual chlamydia screening of all sexually active women younger than 25 years as well as older women with risk factors, such as new or multiple sex partners or a sex partner who has a sexually transmitted infection

- Annual gonorrhea screening for all sexually active women younger than 25 years as well as older women with risk factors, such as new or multiple sex partners or a sex partner who has a sexually transmitted infection

- Syphilis, HIV, chlamydia, and hepatitis B screening for all pregnant women and gonorrhea screening for at-risk pregnant women starting early in pregnancy, with repeat testing as needed, to protect the health of mothers and their infants

- Screening at least once a year for syphilis, chlamydia, and gonorrhea for all sexually active gay, bisexual, and other men who have sex with men (MSM). MSM who have multiple or anonymous partners should be screened more frequently for STDs (ie, at 3- to 6-month intervals).

- Anyone who has unsafe sex or shares injection drug equipment should be tested for HIV at least once a year. Sexually active gay and bisexual men may benefit from more frequent testing (eg, every 3–6 months).

From Workowski KA, Berman S, Centers for Disease Control and Prevention (CDC). Sexually transmitted diseases treatment guidelines, 2010. MMWR Recomm Rep 2010;59(RR-12):1–110.

Combined Hormonal Contraception (Pills, Patches, and Rings)

Overall, the rate of elevated blood pressures in reproductive age women is low. Prior to initiation of CHC, however, blood pressure screening should be performed because estrogen-containing methods are contraindicated for women with hypertension. There is evidence in case-control studies to suggest that women who did not have their blood pressures measured prior to initiation of combined oral contraceptives (COCs) had worse cardiovascular outcomes, including higher risks of myocardial infarction and ischemic stroke.[33–35]

Although it is not required, generally, it is useful to document a baseline weight and body mass index (BMI) to monitor any weight changes that a woman may associate with use of contraception. Obesity, however, is not a contraindication to use of any of the contraceptive methods. Apart from the tests and examinations discussed previously, there are no data to suggest that any other laboratory tests or examinations should be routinely performed prior to initiation of contraceptive methods. Glucose screening, lipid tests, liver enzymes, screening for thrombogenic mutations, Pap smears, and HIV tests are not mandatory prior to initiation. Additionally, no data exist to suggest routine clinical breast examinations are necessary before starting a contraceptive method.

FOLLOW-UP

Routine follow-up is not required after initiation of a contraceptive method because studies have not shown that these visits improve rates of correct or continued use. Providers often require women to return for a string check with an IUD, but this is not required for asymptomatic women. All women should be counseled at the time of initiation to return to clinic at any time to discuss side effects or if they desire to change or discontinue a contraceptive method. In practice, there are certain subpopulations, such as adolescents and women, with multiple medical issues who may benefit from more frequent follow-up. If a follow-up or routine visit occurs, then the provider should take that opportunity to assess a woman's satisfaction with her method and any concerns or side effects. Any changes in medications and medical conditions should be noted and eligibility for the specific method used should be reviewed.

Monitoring for weight changes is beneficial when counseling women who relate weight gain to their contraception. In particular, certain subgroups of women using DMPA may actually experience associated weight gain. One study suggests that already obese adolescent girls have greater weight gain over 18 months of DMPA use compared with girls nonobese at baseline.[36] Another study indicates that adolescents who gain more than 5% of their baseline weight after 6 months of DMPA use are at higher risk for continued weight gain at 12 and 18 months.[37] Because weight gain in the initial few months of use may be predictive of future weight gain, it is important for providers to identify these women early on and provide appropriate counseling and information on alternative methods.

SUMMARY

Providers play an essential role in helping women navigate the many options of contraception that are now available, but they can also create unnecessary barriers. By providing a straightforward and concise set of general guidelines, the SPR can guide providers to safely and effectively initiate contraceptive methods while accounting for each woman's unique circumstances. These evidence-based guidelines serve to prevent providers from performing unnecessary tests and examinations as well as limit delays in initiation of contraception for reasons that are not indicated.

REFERENCES

1. Centers for Disease Control and Prevention (CDC). U S. Medical Eligibility Criteria for Contraceptive Use, 2010. MMWR Recomm Rep 2010;59(RR-4):1–86.
2. Division of Reproductive Health, National Center for Chronic Disease Prevention and Health Promotion, Centers for Disease Control and Prevention (CDC). U.S. Selected Practice Recommendations for Contraceptive Use, 2013: adapted from the World Health Organization Selected Practice Recommendations for Contraceptive Use, 2nd Edition. MMWR Recomm Rep 2013;62(RR-05):1–60.
3. Centers for Disease Control and Prevention (CDC). U S. medical eligibility criteria for contraceptive use. 2010. Available at: http://www.cdc.gov/mmwr/preview/mmwrhtml/rr59e0528a1.htm.
4. Cole LA, Khanlian SA, Sutton JM, et al. Accuracy of home pregnancy tests at the time of missed menses. Am J Obstet Gynecol 2004;190(1):100–5.
5. Wilcox AJ, Baird DD, Dunson D, et al. Natural limits of pregnancy testing in relation to the expected menstrual period. JAMA 2001;286(14):1759–61.
6. Steier JA, Bergsjø P, Myking OL. Human chorionic gonadotropin in maternal plasma after induced abortion, spontaneous abortion, and removed ectopic pregnancy. Obstet Gynecol 1984;64(3):391–4.
7. Korhonen J, Alfthan H, Ylöstalo P, et al. Disappearance of Human Chorionic Gonadotropin and Its Alpha- and Beta-Subunits after Term Pregnancy. Clin Chem 1997;43(11):2155–63.
8. Division of Reproductive Health, National Center for Chronic Disease Prevention and Health Promotion, Centers for Disease Control and Prevention (CDC). U.S. Selected Practice Recommendations for Contraceptive Use. 2013. Available at: http://www.cdc.gov/mmwr/preview/mmwrhtml/rr6205a1.htm?s_cid=rr6205a1_w.
9. Lopez LM, Newmann SJ, Grimes DA, et al. Immediate Start of Hormonal Contraceptives for Contraception. Cochrane Database Syst Rev 2012;(12):CD006260.
10. Whiteman MK, Tyler CP, Folger SG, et al. When can a woman have an intrauterine device inserted? A systematic review. Contraception 2013;87(5):666–73.
11. Brahmi D, Curtis KM. When can a woman start combined hormonal contraceptives (CHCs)? A systematic review. Contraception 2013;87(5):524–38.
12. Lopez LM, Newmann SJ, Grimes DA, et al. Immediate Start of Hormonal Contraceptives for Contraception. Cochrane Database Syst Rev 2008;(2):CD006260. The Cochrane Collaboration (Chichester, UK: John Wiley & Sons, Ltd, 2008).
13. Westhoff C, Heartwell S, Edwards S, et al. Initiation of oral contraceptives using a quick start compared with a conventional start: a randomized controlled trial. Obstet Gynecol 2007;109(6):1270–6.
14. Kapp N, Gaffield ME. Initiation of progestogen-only injectables on different days of the menstrual cycle and its effect on contraceptive effectiveness and compliance: a systematic review. Contraception 2013;87(5):576–82.
15. Jellesen R, Strandberg-Larsen K, Jørgensen T, et al. Maternal use of oral contraceptives and risk of fetal death. Paediatr Perinat Epidemiol 2008;22(4):334–40.
16. Bracken MB. Oral contraception and congenital malformations in offspring: a review and meta-analysis of the prospective studies. Obstet Gynecol 1990;76(3 Pt 2):552–7.
17. Waller DK, Gallaway MS, Taylor LG, et al. Use of oral contraceptives in pregnancy and major structural birth defects in offspring. Epidemiology 2010;21(2):232–9.
18. Brahmi D, Steenland MW, Renner RM, et al. Pregnancy outcomes with an IUD in situ: a systematic review. Contraception 2012;85(2):131–9.

19. Steenland MW, Rodriguez MI, Marchbanks PA, et al. How does the number of oral contraceptive pill packs dispensed or prescribed affect continuation and other measures of consistent and correct use? A systematic review. Contraception 2013;87(5):605–10.
20. Foster DG, Parvataneni R, de Bocanegra HT, et al. Number of oral contraceptive pill packages dispensed, method continuation, and costs. Obstet Gynecol 2006; 108(5):1107–14.
21. White KO, Westhoff C. The effect of pack supply on oral contraceptive pill continuation: a randomized controlled trial. Obstet Gynecol 2011;118(3):615–22.
22. Foster DG, Hulett D, Bradsberry M, et al. Number of oral contraceptive pill packages dispensed and subsequent unintended pregnancies. Obstet Gynecol 2011;117(3):566–72.
23. Canto De Cetina TE, Canto P, Ordoñez Luna M. Effect of counseling to improve compliance in mexican women receiving depot-medroxyprogesterone acetate. Contraception 2001;63(3):143–6.
24. Lei ZW, Wu SC, Garceau RJ, et al. Effect of pretreatment counseling on discontinuation rates in chinese women given depo-medroxyprogesterone acetate for contraception. Contraception 1996;53(6):357–61.
25. Speroff L, Mishell DR. The postpartum visit: it's time for a change in order to optimally initiate contraception. Contraception 2008;78(2):90–8.
26. King J. Contraception and Lactation. J Midwifery Womens Health 2007;52(6): 614–20.
27. Kapp N, Curtis KM. Combined oral contraceptive use among breastfeeding women: a systematic review. Contraception 2010;82(1):10–6.
28. Lopez LM, Grey TW, Stuebe AM, et al. Combined Hormonal versus Nonhormonal versus Progestin-Only Contraception in Lactation. Cochrane Database Syst Rev 2015;(3):CD003988.
29. Sonalkar S, Kapp N. Intrauterine device insertion in the postpartum period: a systematic review. Eur J Contracept Reprod Health Care 2015;20(1):4–18.
30. Chen BA, Reeves MF, Hayes JL, et al. Postplacental or delayed insertion of the levonorgestrel intrauterine device after vaginal delivery: a randomized controlled trial. Obstet Gynecol 2010;116(5):1079–87.
31. Gaffield ME, Kapp N, Ravi A. Use of combined oral contraceptives post abortion. Contraception 2009;80(4):355–62.
32. Farley TM, Rosenberg MJ, Rowe PJ, et al. Intrauterine devices and pelvic inflammatory disease: an international perspective. Lancet 1992;339(8796):785–8.
33. Tepper NK, Curtis KM, Steenland MW, et al. Blood pressure measurement prior to initiating hormonal contraception: a systematic review. Contraception 2013;87(5): 631–8.
34. Acute Myocardial Infarction and Combined Oral Contraceptives: Results of an International Multicentre Case-Control Study. WHO Collaborative Study of Cardiovascular Disease and Steroid Hormone Contraception. Lancet 1997;349(9060):1202–9.
35. Ischaemic Stroke and Combined Oral Contraceptives: Results of an International, Multicentre, Case-Control Study. WHO Collaborative Study of Cardiovascular Disease and Steroid Hormone Contraception. Lancet 1996;348(9026):498–505.
36. Bonny AE, Ziegler J, Harvey R, et al. Weight gain in obese and nonobese adolescent girls initiating depot medroxyprogesterone, oral contraceptive pills, or no hormonal contraceptive method. Arch Pediatr Adolesc Med 2006;160(1):40–5.
37. Bonny AE, Secic M, Cromer B. Early weight gain related to later weight gain in adolescents on depot medroxyprogesterone acetate. Obstet Gynecol 2011; 117(4):793–7.

Why Stop Now? Extended and Continuous Regimens of Combined Hormonal Contraceptive Methods

Lyndsey S. Benson, MD, MS*, Elizabeth A. Micks, MD, MPH

KEYWORDS

- Combined hormonal contraception • Combined oral contraceptive pills
- Extended contraceptive use • Continuous contraceptive use
- Ovulation suppression • Bleeding profile with contraception
- Contraceptive vaginal ring • Contraceptive transdermal patch

KEY POINTS

Extended and continuous combined hormonal regimens result in:

- Decreased frequency of scheduled bleeding.
- Initial increase in unscheduled bleeding that lessens over time.
- Decrease in estrogen-withdrawal symptoms and improved control of medical conditions.
- Likely improved efficacy due to more consistent ovulation suppression.
- High user acceptability.

INTRODUCTION

Combined oral contraceptives (COCs) are the most common reversible birth control used by US women, a fact that has remained unchanged over several decades despite the introduction of many new contraceptive methods.[1] More than one in four women in the United States using contraception is using COCs.[1] Thirty percent of women in the United States are currently using some form of combined hormonal contraception (CHC) as their method of contraception, including COCs, the transdermal patch, and the vaginal ring.[1] Four out of every five sexually experienced women in the United States have used COCs.[2]

Since their initial introduction more than 50 years ago, COCs traditionally have been prescribed in 28-day cycles. COCs were designed to mimic the menstrual cycle with

Department of Obstetrics and Gynecology, University of Washington, 1959 Northeast Pacific Street, Box 356460, Seattle, WA 98195, USA
* Corresponding author.
E-mail address: lsbenson@uw.edu

Obstet Gynecol Clin N Am 42 (2015) 669–681
http://dx.doi.org/10.1016/j.ogc.2015.07.009
0889-8545/15/$ – see front matter © 2015 Elsevier Inc. All rights reserved.

21 active hormone pills followed by seven placebo pills resulting in a regular withdrawal bleed every 28 days. Changes to dose, progestin and estrogen formulation, and regimens have been made over the years to improve the efficacy, bleeding profile, safety, and tolerability associated with CHCs.

Many women desire a decreased frequency in menstrual cycles.[3,4] Decreasing the number of withdrawal bleeds per year may improve women's quality of life by decreasing menstrual and premenstrual symptoms resulting in fewer days of missed work or school and reducing the cost of sanitary supplies. Women may also prefer not to have a withdrawal bleed for social and cultural reasons.[5,6] Additionally, changes to traditional CHC regimens improve side effect profiles, increase ovulation suppression, and decrease unintended pregnancy rates. This article explores extended and continuous CHC regimens including efficacy, safety, bleeding profiles, and management of other gynecologic conditions.

DEFINITIONS

Terminology used in the discussion of CHC regimens is inconsistent. In this article, we use "traditional regimen" to refer to CHCs prescribed in a 28-day cycle (**Table 1**). These traditional cyclic regimens typically include 21 days of active hormones with 7 days of placebo, allowing for a withdrawal bleed each cycle. "Traditional regimens with shortened hormone-free interval" refer to 28-day regimens with less than 7 hormone-free days each cycle. Food and Drug Administration (FDA)-approved regimens include 24/4 and 26/2 regimens. Some clinicians and researchers use the term "extended regimen" to refer to any regimen with more than 21 days of active hormones, including the 24/4 and 26/2 regimens. However, in the context of this article, we define extended regimen as any regimen where active hormones are used for longer than 28 days, with a scheduled hormone-free interval, or an interval with decreased hormones with the intent of having a withdrawal bleed less frequently than every 28 days.

The common FDA-approved extended regimens are designed as 84/7 regimens, meaning women can expect one scheduled withdrawal bleed every 3 months. Variations on the extended regimen include tailored and flexible extended regimens.

Table 1 Definitions	
Term	**Description**
Traditional regimen	28-d cycle with 21 active hormone days and 7 placebo days
Traditional regimen with shortened hormone-free interval	28-d regimen with <7 hormone-free days each cycle (eg, 24/4 regimens)
Extended regimen	Active hormones taken continuously for longer than 28 d followed by a hormone-free or decreased hormone interval
Flexible extended regimen	Extended regimens with user-initiated hormone-free intervals either because of bleeding or user preference
Tailored extended regimen	Extended regimens with hormone-free intervals triggered by unscheduled bleeding/spotting
Continuous regimen	Regimens taken in an uninterrupted fashion with no hormone-free interval

"Flexible extended regimens" refer to extended regimens where the user initiates hormone-free intervals either because of bleeding or for user preference. "Tailored extended regimens" refer to extended regimens with hormone-free intervals triggered by breakthrough bleeding or spotting. "Continuous regimens" then refer to COCs designed to be taken in an uninterrupted fashion with no hormone-free interval.

DEVELOPMENT OF EXTENDED AND CONTINUOUS REGIMEN

The bleeding that occurs with traditional CHC regimens is not medically necessary. The scheduled hormone-free interval and associated withdrawal bleeding was designed for cultural and religious reasons, not for any physiologic necessity. Currently, many women desire decreased menstrual bleeding and frequency, which makes elimination of the hormone-free interval an attractive option.[4,7] Newer COC formulations have been developed over the past several decades to improve tolerability and bleeding profiles, using variable estrogen or progestin types and doses, and shortened or absent hormone-free intervals. Extended and continuous regimens decrease or eliminate scheduled withdrawal bleeds, but also increase the amount of unscheduled bleeding and spotting, at least initially. Improved bleeding profile and other benefits of COCs may increase patient satisfaction, compliance, and continuation, factors that contribute to contraceptive efficacy. This is a critical research priority, because the typical use failure rate for all CHCs is 9% per year.[8] Continuation rates are currently low for CHCs; they are significantly lower than that of long-term reversible methods including the intrauterine device and contraceptive implant.[9]

Traditional cyclic COC regimens continue to be used widely. However, extended regimens have been explored since the 1970s.[10] The first COC designed specifically for extended use, with ethinyl estradiol (EE), 30 µg, and levonorgestrel (LNG), 150 µg, for 84 consecutive days followed by seven inert pills, was approved by the FDA in 2003 (Seasonale). Since then, a variety of brand-name and generic extended-regimen COCs have entered the market (**Table 2**). Newer formulations have replaced the hormone-free interval with low-dose estrogen pills (10 µg EE) to improve ovulation suppression and decrease symptoms related to hormone withdrawal (Seasonique,

Table 2
FDA-approved extended and continuous regimens

Brand	Generic	Regimen
Seasonale (Teva)	Jolessa (Teva) Quasense (Actavis) Introvale (Sandoz)	84 d: 150 µg LNG + 30 µg EE 7 d: placebo
Seasonique (Teva)	Amethia (Actavis) Camrese (Teva) Ashlyna (Glenmark) Daysee (Lupin)	84 d: 150 µg LNG + 30 µg EE 7 d: 10 µg EE
LoSeasonique (Teva)	Amethia Lo (Actavis) Camrese Lo (Teva)	84 d: 100 µg LNG + 20 µg EE 7 d: 10 µg EE
Quartette (Teva)	—	42 d: 150 µg LNG + 20 µg EE 21 d: 150 µg LNG + 25 µg EE 21 d: 150 µg LNG + 30 µg EE 7 d: 10 µg EE
Lybrel[a] (Wyeth)	Amethyst (Actavis)	Continuous: 90 µg LNG + 20 µg EE

[a] Discontinued by manufacturer.

LoSeasonique). There is one FDA-approved continuous pill (Lybrel) comprised of EE, 20 µg, and LNG, 90 µg, which has been available since 2007. However, in practice providers often prescribe traditional cyclic COCs and offer women the option of discarding the placebo pills and using active pills continuously. The downside of this practice is that women often have to go to the pharmacy every 3 weeks instead of every 4 weeks to obtain a new pill pack and certain insurance plans may restrict how frequently women can obtain pill packs.

For more than two decades, trials of extended-regimen COCs have been associated with frequent unscheduled bleeding and spotting.[11] Pharmaceutical companies have developed several new options to address this problem (see **Table 2**). A more recent attempt to reduce unscheduled bleeding observed with extended COCs is the introduction of the ascending-dose extended regimen. The first FDA-approved ascending-dose extended-regimen COC, Quartette, is divided into 91-day cycles that include LNG for 84 days combined with 20 µg EE for 42 days, 25 µg EE for 21 days, and 30 µg EE for 21 days, followed by 7 days of 10 µg EE alone.[12] The ascending-dose extended regimen increases EE dose at the times in the cycle when unscheduled bleeding is most likely, while minimizing EE exposure overall. However, there is no evidence that reduction of EE dose below 30 µg is associated with improved safety. Given the favorable bleeding profile over time of the low estrogen dose extended regimen (LoSeasonique), it remains to be seen in future studies whether the ascending-dose extended-regimen approach offers any additional benefits.[13]

EFFICACY

Despite perfect use failure rates of 0.3% for CHCs, typical use rates are estimated to be 9%.[8] Typical use failure rates are higher primarily because of user error or noncompliance, including missed or delayed pills. CHCs work through several mechanisms, primarily thickening of the cervical mucus and suppression of ovulation. The greatest risk of method failure occurs at the end of the placebo period, when the risk of ovulation can be amplified by a delay in starting the next active pills. With older COCs containing significantly higher doses of hormones than current formulations, a longer placebo period was required before serum hormone concentrations would decrease enough to elicit a withdrawal bleed. Current formulations with lower doses of estrogens have resulted in a shorter onset to withdrawal bleed, and a higher probability of rising follicle-stimulating hormone and ovulation by the end of a 7-day hormone-free interval.

Shortening the hormone-free interval in 24/4 regimens has been shown to improve ovarian suppression, thereby decreasing the risk of ovulation during the placebo period.[14] Extended and continuous regimens may yield a further improvement in ovulation suppression. Birch and colleagues[15] showed that continuous regimens effectively prevented development of dominant follicles in a trial randomizing 36 women to traditional versus continuous COC use.

Theoretically, an improvement in ovulation suppression translates to improved efficacy and decreased unintended pregnancy rates. Prospective COC trials are typically not powered to detect differences in unintended pregnancies between regimens, given that the numbers of unintended pregnancies occurring in these trials are so low. However, Dinger and colleagues[16] were able to compare contraceptive failure rates for 24/4 and 21/7 regimens using outcome data from 52,218 US participants in the International Active Surveillance of Women Taking Oral Contraceptives cohort study. They found a lower contraceptive failure rate in women taking COCs with a shortened hormone-free interval, although failure rates were low overall, with an estimated failure of 2.1% for 24/4 drospirenone-EE compared with 2.8% for 21/7 drospirenone-EE.[16] Given the improved efficacy associated with traditional regimens with a shortened hormone-free interval, presumably secondary to improved ovulation suppression and compliance, we would expect that extended and continuous regimens may demonstrate further improvement.

In a recent Cochrane review, Edelman and colleagues[17] found no significant difference in number of pregnancies with traditional versus continuous or extended regimens in most trials examined. The one exception was a study from 1995 by Coutinho and colleagues[18] that randomized 900 women to continuous versus traditional cyclic use of a vaginally administered combined hormonal pill; there were four unintended pregnancies, all of which occurred in the traditional regimen arm. A more recent study by Anderson and colleagues[19] found that pregnancy rates over 1 year were 0.9% for an extended regimen versus 1.3% for a traditional regimen, although this difference was not statistically significant.

A retrospective claims study demonstrated significantly lower pregnancy rates among women taking 84/7 regimens compared with 21/7 (4.4% vs 7.3%; $P<.0001$) and 24/4 regimens (4.4% vs 6.9%; $P<.0001$) over 1 year.[20] However, this study was limited because indication for COC use was not available in the claims database, and women taking extended regimens may have been more likely to be using the COC for noncontraceptive purposes (eg, dysmenorrhea or heavy menstrual bleeding).

Overall effectiveness of a contraceptive method depends not only on efficacy of the method itself (ie, success of ovulation suppression when comparing extended and continuous regimens with traditional regimens), but also on women's compliance with, and continuation of, a given method. Edelman and colleagues[17] looked at continuation rates and adherence in their Cochrane review. Most included studies (11 of 13) reported no difference in continuation rates between traditional regimens and extended or continuous regimens. Two trials did report higher discontinuation in the extended- or continuous-regimen arms. For example, Anderson and Hait[19] reported that only 59.4% of extended-regimen patients completed 1 year of use, compared with 71.2% of patients in the traditional-regimen arm. Participant adherence was reported in five of the trials included in the Cochrane review; no significant differences were seen between arms in any of those studies.[17]

In summary, extended and continuous regimens are associated with improved ovarian suppression and seem to improve contraceptive efficacy compared with traditional regimens. Additionally, fewer hormone-free intervals may simplify COC regimens by decreasing opportunities for delay in starting subsequent pill packs. Continuous regimens in particular may improve patient adherence simply because there is less room for error when taking the same pill with the same hormone dosage each day.

SAFETY

Venous thromboembolism (VTE) risk is increased with use of CHCs, particularly in the first year, and risk seems to be related to estrogen dose. Older regimens with EE doses 50 μg or greater are associated with higher risk of VTE compared with 10- to 30-μg regimens; there is no evidence that reductions in EE dose below 30 μg result in a further decrease in VTE risk.[21,22] A theoretic increase in VTE risk has been suggested with extended and continuous regimens because of increased exposure to estrogen, although none of these regimens contain more than 30 μg EE daily. The recent Cochrane review by Edelman and colleagues[17] reviewed adverse event data in 12 randomized trials. There were no adverse events in 10 of the trials. In the remaining two trials, one woman using an extended regimen in each study experienced a thromboembolic event; each of these women had risk factors other than their COC regimens.[19,23] There is no evidence that extended or continuous COC regimens are associated with a significant increase in thromboembolic events, or any other adverse events, compared with traditional regimens.

In women who are not using hormonal contraception, absence of menses is a major risk factor for endometrial hyperplasia and malignancy. However, in women using any hormonal method of contraception, there is no evidence that withdrawal bleeding is medically necessary. The progestin component of CHCs seems to maintain a thin and inactive endometrial lining. Although hormone withdrawal reliably leads to uterine bleeding during the hormone-free interval, there is no physiologic need for endometrial shedding. Four studies included in the recent Cochrane review specifically monitored endometrial safety. No differences between the extended regimens and traditional regimens were noted. Anderson and colleagues[24] reviewed paired endometrial biopsies obtained from 63 subjects before and after use of Seasonique for 1 year to determine whether the replacement of the hormone-free interval with low-dose estrogen had any untoward effects on the endometrium. No increase in endometrial pathology was noted and a rapid return to normal cycling endometrium occurred following discontinuation of the extended regimen.

Additionally, fertility is not delayed following use of extended and continuous COC regimens. Anderson and colleagues[25] monitored 189 women using an extended-regimen for 2 years and found no delay in return to fertility even after long-term use.

BLEEDING PROFILE

Unscheduled or breakthrough bleeding is the most commonly reported side effect with extended or continuous COC regimens. In general, extended and continuous CHC regimens decrease scheduled bleeding episodes at the expense of an initial increase in unscheduled bleeding and spotting. The FDA-approved extended COC regimens decrease scheduled withdrawal bleeding to once every 3 months, whereas continuous COC regimens eliminate scheduled withdrawal bleeds altogether. Studies evaluating bleeding profile with COCs use inconsistent terminology, but researchers are increasingly using World Health Organization definitions of bleeding (requiring sanitary protection) and spotting (light bleeding that does not require the use of sanitary protection). Of note, there do not seem to be any trials directly comparing bleeding profiles with traditional regimens versus traditional regimens with shortened hormone-free intervals.

Edelman and colleagues[17] reviewed 11 trials in which women were randomized to traditional CHC regimens versus extended or continuous regimens with a primary outcome of bleeding profile. Most trials demonstrated either no difference in overall bleeding days or fewer days of bleeding and/or spotting with the extended and continuous regimens.

Anderson and Hait[19] randomized 682 women to extended (84/7) versus traditional regimens of 150 µg LNG and 30 µg EE. They found that women receiving the 84/7 extended regimen experienced decreased bleeding days (35 vs 53 days over 1 year of use). They found an initial increase in unscheduled bleeding with the extended regimen, but the number of unscheduled bleeding days decreased each cycle and was comparable with unscheduled bleeding seen with the traditional regimen by the fourth extended cycle. Miller and Hughes[26] also demonstrated an increase in spotting days with a continuous COC regimen versus a traditional regimen, but after 9 months the continuous COC arm was reporting fewer spotting days than the traditional arm.

In a phase 3 evaluation of a continuous regimen of 90 µg LNG and 20 µg EE, 18.5% of the 2134 enrolled subjects discontinued for reasons related to the bleeding profile.[27] One study suggests that increasing the EE content in a continuous COC regimen from 20 µg to 30 µg does not have an apparent benefit in terms of bleeding profile.[28]

Rates of amenorrhea also increase as the duration of an extended or continuous COC regimen increases. In the Miller and Hughes[26] study, complete amenorrhea was noted by 16% of women in the continuous regimen arm during the first 3 months, and increased to 72% by cycles 10 to 12. For women using a continuous COC for 2 years, amenorrhea rates increased further from 63.6% at the end of the first year to 80.7% at the end of the second year.[29] Including women with only spotting in addition to complete amenorrhea, these numbers increase to 87% and 94.7%, respectively.

TREATMENT OF MENSTRUAL SYMPTOMS AND OTHER MEDICAL CONDITIONS

Women who have cyclic symptoms benefit from extended and continuous use of COCs. Edelman and coworkers[17] reported a decrease in dysmenorrhea, headaches, and nausea in several of the studies included in their Cochrane review.

Dmitrovic and colleagues[30] randomized 29 women with primary dysmenorrhea to continuous versus traditional 21/7 regimens of 75 µg gestodene and 20 µg EE. They found an improvement in pain scores with continuous COCs at the end of 1 and 3 months, and a trend toward lower pain scores in the continuous arm at the end of the 6-month study.

Continuous COC regimens are frequently used as treatment of endometriosis, especially in the postoperative period. Vercellini and colleagues[31] noted a significant improvement in pain scores with use of a continuous COC regimen for women who had surgery for endometriosis followed by recurrent symptoms while on a traditional COC regimen. Fifty women who experienced recurrent dysmenorrhea while on traditional regimen COCs following surgery for endometriosis were switched to a continuous COC in this prospective, self-controlled trial. Mean pain scores decreased from 75 ± 13 with the traditional regimen to 31 ± 17 with the continuous regimen ($P<.001$). A recent systematic review found that continuous COCs were superior to traditional regimens following conservative surgical management of endometriosis.[32] The authors reviewed four studies and found decreased recurrence of dysmenorrhea, nonspecific pelvic pain, and endometriomas in women taking COCs in a continuous fashion.

PATIENT ACCEPTABILITY

Most women desire a decreased frequency in menstrual bleeding. Nonetheless, most randomized trials included in the 2014 Cochrane review found no significant improvement in patient satisfaction with extended and continuous regimens.[17] Satisfaction ratings in these studies were high overall, with most women in extended/continuous and traditional regimen arms reporting that they were satisfied with their method. Six months after the conclusion of a 1-year extended COC regimen study, most participants had continued on the extended regimen.[33]

Several trials have demonstrated a higher discontinuation rate with extended and continuous COC regimens because of unscheduled bleeding. Five randomized trials included in the recent Cochrane review reported that a greater number of subjects in the extended or continuous arms discontinued because of bleeding problems, whereas no difference was noted in the remaining seven trials.[17] As described previously, a phase 3 evaluation of a continuous COC regimen by Archer and colleagues[27] demonstrated an 18.5% discontinuation rate for reasons related to the bleeding profile.

FLEXIBLE AND TAILORED REGIMENS

The initial increase in unscheduled bleeding and spotting is a significant downside to extended and continuous regimens. Women initiating these regimens must be counseled that the bleeding profile typically improves within the first 6 months to 1 year of use. A novel approach involves altering or adjusting the timing of the hormone-free interval to improve the bleeding profile. According to the Centers for Disease Control and Prevention Selected Practice Recommendations for Contraceptive Use, women using COCs continuously may choose to initiate a hormone-free interval for 3 to 4 days whenever they have 3 or more consecutive days of bleeding (with the requirement that they have taken active hormone pills for at least the previous 21 days continuously).[34]

A tailored extended regimen refers to an extended CHC regimen where a hormone-free interval is initiated when unscheduled bleeding occurs. In a study of 111 women using an extended COC regimen, women who experienced 7 consecutive days of unscheduled bleeding or spotting were randomized to continuation of active pills versus initiation of a hormone-free interval for 3 days. Forty-eight (47%) of the participants experienced a total of 63 eligible bleeding events, which were randomized individually. The initiation of a 3-day hormone-free interval was significantly more effective in resolving the current bleeding episode ($P<.0001$).[35]

A large clinical trial by Jensen and colleagues[36] randomized 1887 women to either a tailored extended regimen (hormone-free interval triggered by 3 days of unscheduled bleeding/spotting), a flexible extended regimen (hormone-free interval could be initiated at any time, independent of the occurrence of bleeding), or a 24/4 regimen of 3 mg drospirenone and 20 μg EE. They found that women who initiated 4-day hormone-free intervals following 3 days of unscheduled bleeding had the lowest number of mean bleeding and spotting days over a 1-year period (40 days for the tailored extended regimen vs 47 days and 52 days for the flexible extended regimen and the conventional 24/4 regimen, respectively). All three regimens were well-tolerated and pregnancy rates were low overall (1.63% cumulative pregnancy rate at the end of 1 year). User satisfaction was high in all three arms, with 77%, 70%, and 76% of women using the tailored extended regimen, the flexible extended regimen, and the conventional 24/4 regimen reporting that they were "very much" or "much" satisfied, respectively. Most women (95% in the tailored extended regimen arm and 98% in the flexible extended regimen arm) believed that instructions for each regimen were easy to understand. Additionally, no significant differences in adverse events or discontinuation rates were noted between the three arms. A phase 3, multicenter trial was conducted in which 755 women continued on a tailored extended regimen of 3 mg drospirenone and 20 μg EE for a second year.[37] This regimen remained well-tolerated with a favorable safety profile over 2 years.

NON-ORAL COMBINED HORMONAL CONTRACEPTIVES

Most trials looking at alternatives to traditional CHC regimens, including the trials discussed previously, focus on oral contraceptive pills. COCs are the most popular CHC, with 17.1%, 0.5%, and 1.3% of all US women using the pill, patch, and ring, respectively.[1] However, 10% of women have used the patch at some point in their lifetimes and 6% have ever used the ring.[2] Extended or continuous use of these methods is an active area of investigation.

Guazzelli and colleagues[38] examined extended regimen use of the etonorgestrel/EE vaginal ring in a prospective cohort of 150 women. They found that women who used either the ring or COCs in an 84/7 extended regimen experienced a significant reduction in scheduled and unscheduled bleeding over the course of 1 year. Another study randomized 429 women to four different regimens of the contraceptive vaginal ring: 28-day, 49-day, 91-day, and 364-day cycles.[23] However, women in the extended and continuous arms were more likely to discontinue early ($P = .017$ and $P = .005$, respectively), primarily for bleeding-related reasons. The easiest way to instruct women on continuous use of the ring is simply to remove and replace the ring on the same calendar day each month.

The vaginal ring can also be used in a tailored extended regimen. In one prospective trial, 65 women were randomized to use the ring continuously (replacing it on the same calendar day each month with no ring-free days) versus a tailored extended regimen where women initiated a 4-day hormone-free interval if they experienced 5 consecutive bleeding days.[39] Women using the latter method experienced a greater number of days without breakthrough bleeding or spotting (95% vs 89%; $P = .016$) over the course of 6 months.

Few studies have examined extended or continuous use of the norelgestromin/EE transdermal patch. Stewart and colleagues[40] randomized 239 women to use the patch in a traditional 21/7 versus an extended 84/7 regimen for 16 weeks total. Extended patch users experienced fewer bleeding and spotting days, and satisfaction was high in both groups. However, there are some concerns regarding extended or continuous patch use because of increasing serum EE levels over time before the patch-free week.[41] It is hoped that ongoing studies regarding the pharmacokinetics of extended patch use will clarify any increased risk with extended or continuous patch use versus COC and vaginal ring regimens. For now, there is no clear evidence to support or refute claims that extended or continuous use of the patch versus other CHCs may be associated with increased risk of VTE or other adverse events.

SUMMARY

Despite the evidence regarding the safety and efficacy of extended and continuous regimens, these approaches are underused. A survey of women's health care providers demonstrated that most (73.5%) continue to prescribe traditional regimens most commonly.[42] Eighteen percent of the 799 health care providers surveyed thought extended use of COCs was associated with one or more health problems, including increased risk of breast cancer, VTE, or future fertility problems.

Extended and continuous regimens are safe and effective, with high user satisfaction. Growing epidemiologic evidence and clear biologic plausibility suggest that extended and continuous regimens may prevent pregnancy more effectively than traditional cyclic regimens because of improved ovulation suppression. Women also appreciate the ability to decrease the frequency of scheduled bleeding. The new flexible and tailored regimens mean that the regimen can be individualized to each woman, allowing her more control over the bleeding profile. Although there is typically an initial increase in unscheduled bleeding, this resolves after several months. Users of continuous CHC regimens experience an increasing rate of amenorrhea over time.

Women are individuals, and different women want different things out of their contraceptive methods. CHCs are significantly less effective than long-acting methods yet they continue to be popular among patients and health care providers, likely because they are simple to prescribe and use and are started and stopped without a separate clinic visit. All women choosing CHCs should be counseled regarding the option of

---

Box 1
Tips for counseling women regarding extended or continuous use of CHCs

- There is no medical reason for cyclic withdrawal bleeding while taking hormonal contraception
- Expect an increase in unscheduled bleeding, especially over the first 3–6 months of use
- Unscheduled bleeding may be improved by initiating a 3- to 4-day hormone-free interval following at least 21 days of continuous use
- Higher rates of amenorrhea
- Easier to remember and likely more effective
- Same return to fertility if you decide to become pregnant
- COCs and the ring are safe for extended and continuous use

---

extended and continuous regimens. Contraceptive users should be encouraged to make an informed decision and be provided with reasonable expectations regarding bleeding profiles. Additionally, health care providers should recommend tailored extended regimens as an intervention for unscheduled bleeding. Women using continuous methods can easily follow instructions to initiate a 3- to 5-day hormone-free interval whenever 3 or more consecutive bleeding days are experienced, assuming it has been at least 24 days since the last hormone-free interval.

COC users can be prescribed an FDA-approved extended or continuous regimen. Any monophasic traditional 21/7 regimen COC can also be prescribed in an extended or continuous fashion with instructions to skip 1 or more placebo week. Downsides to this approach include limitations in obtaining more than one pill pack per month and remembering off-label instructions. Multiphasic COCs, including newer ascending-dose extended regimens, do not have any proven benefit. The contraceptive vaginal ring can be used in an extended or continuous manner. Continuous ring users can simply remove and replace the ring on the same calendar day each month, making this an optimal method for women interested in decreasing or eliminating scheduled withdrawal bleeds. Extended or continuous use of the contraceptive transdermal patch should not be encouraged for the general population until more data are available regarding pharmacokinetics and safety profile.

Extended and continuous regimens give women the opportunity to decrease withdrawal bleeding at the expense of a short-term increase in unscheduled bleeding/spotting. These regimens can also suppress ovulation more consistently, decrease estrogen-withdrawal symptoms, and improve control of other medical conditions. All women choosing CHCs should be counseled regarding the potential benefits of extended and continuous regimens compared with traditional cyclic regimens (**Box 1**). The time has come to move beyond the constraints of the traditional 21/7 COC regimen.

REFERENCES

1. Jones J, Mosher W, Daniels K. Current contraceptive use in the United States, 2006-2010, and changes in patterns of use since 1995. Natl Health Stat Rep 2012;(60):1–25.
2. Daniels K, Mosher WD. Contraceptive methods women have ever used: United States, 1982-2010. Natl Health Stat Rep 2013;(62):1–15.

3. den Tonkelaar I, Oddens BJ. Preferred frequency and characteristics of menstrual bleeding in relation to reproductive status, oral contraceptive use, and hormone replacement therapy use. Contraception 1999;59(6):357–62.

4. Edelman A, Lew R, Cwiak C, et al. Acceptability of contraceptive-induced amenorrhea in a racially diverse group of US women. Contraception 2007;75(6):450–3.

5. Cote I, Jacobs P, Cumming D. Work loss associated with increased menstrual loss in the United States. Obstet Gynecol 2002;100(4):683–7.

6. Schwartz JL, Creinin MD, Pymar HC. The trimonthly combination oral contraceptive regimen: is it cost effective? Contraception 1999;60(5):263–7.

7. Andrist LC, Arias RD, Nucatola D, et al. Women's and providers' attitudes toward menstrual suppression with extended use of oral contraceptives. Contraception 2004;70(5):359–63.

8. Trussell J. Contraceptive failure in the United States. Contraception 2011;83(5):397–404.

9. O'Neil-Callahan M, Peipert JF, Zhao Q, et al. Twenty-four-month continuation of reversible contraception. Obstet Gynecol 2013;122(5):1083–91.

10. Loudon NB, Foxwell M, Potts DM, et al. Acceptability of an oral contraceptive that reduces the frequency of menstruation: the tri-cycle pill regimen. Br Med J 1977;2(6085):487–90.

11. Kaunitz AM. Menstruation: choosing whether... and when. Contraception 2000;62(6):277–84.

12. Portman DJ, Kaunitz AM, Howard B, et al. Efficacy and safety of an ascending-dose, extended-regimen levonorgestrel/ethinyl estradiol combined oral contraceptive. Contraception 2014;89(4):299–306.

13. Krishnan S, Kiley J. The lowest-dose, extended-cycle combined oral contraceptive pill with continuous ethinyl estradiol in the United States: a review of the literature on ethinyl estradiol 20 mug/levonorgestrel 100 mug + ethinyl estradiol 10 mug. Int J Womens Health 2010;2:235–9.

14. Klipping C, Duijkers I, Trummer D, et al. Suppression of ovarian activity with a drospirenone-containing oral contraceptive in a 24/4 regimen. Contraception 2008;78(1):16–25.

15. Birtch RL, Olatunbosun OA, Pierson RA. Ovarian follicular dynamics during conventional vs. continuous oral contraceptive use. Contraception 2006;73(3):235–43.

16. Dinger J, Minh TD, Buttmann N, et al. Effectiveness of oral contraceptive pills in a large U.S. cohort comparing progestogen and regimen. Obstet Gynecol 2011;117(1):33–40.

17. Edelman A, Micks E, Gallo MF, et al. Continuous or extended cycle vs. cyclic use of combined hormonal contraceptives for contraception. Cochrane Database Syst Rev 2014;(7):CD004695.

18. Coutinho EM, O'Dwyer E, Barbosa IC, et al. Comparative study on intermittent versus continuous use of a contraceptive pill administered by vaginal route. Contraception 1995;51(6):355–8.

19. Anderson FD, Hait H. A multicenter, randomized study of an extended cycle oral contraceptive. Contraception 2003;68(2):89–96.

20. Howard B, Trussell J, Grubb E, et al. Comparison of rates of and charges from pregnancy complications in users of extended and cyclic combined oral contraceptive (COC) regimens: a brief report. Contraception 2014;89(5):396–9.

21. de Bastos M, Stegeman BH, Rosendaal FR, et al. Combined oral contraceptives: venous thrombosis. Cochrane Database Syst Rev 2014;(3):CD010813.

22. Inman WH. Monitoring of adverse reactions to drugs in the United Kingdom. Proc R Soc Med 1970;63(12):1302–4.

23. Miller L, Verhoeven CH, Hout J. Extended regimens of the contraceptive vaginal ring: a randomized trial. Obstet Gynecol 2005;106(3):473–82.

24. Anderson FD, Feldman R, Reape KZ. Endometrial effects of a 91-day extended-regimen oral contraceptive with low-dose estrogen in place of placebo. Contraception 2008;77(2):91–6.

25. Anderson FD, Gibbons W, Portman D. Long-term safety of an extended-cycle oral contraceptive (Seasonale): a 2-year multicenter open-label extension trial. Am J Obstet Gynecol 2006;195(1):92–6.

26. Miller L, Hughes JP. Continuous combination oral contraceptive pills to eliminate withdrawal bleeding: a randomized trial. Obstet Gynecol 2003;101(4):653–61.

27. Archer DF, Jensen JT, Johnson JV, et al. Evaluation of a continuous regimen of levonorgestrel/ethinyl estradiol: phase 3 study results. Contraception 2006; 74(6):439–45.

28. Edelman AB, Koontz SL, Nichols MD, et al. Continuous oral contraceptives: are bleeding patterns dependent on the hormones given? Obstet Gynecol 2006; 107(3):657–65.

29. Reid RL, Fortier MP, Smith L, et al. Safety and bleeding profile of continuous levonorgestrel 90 mcg/ethinyl estradiol 20 mcg based on 2 years of clinical trial data in Canada. Contraception 2010;82(6):497–502.

30. Dmitrovic R, Kunselman AR, Legro RS. Continuous compared with cyclic oral contraceptives for the treatment of primary dysmenorrhea: a randomized controlled trial. Obstet Gynecol 2012;119(6):1143–50.

31. Vercellini P, Frontino G, De Giorgi O, et al. Continuous use of an oral contraceptive for endometriosis-associated recurrent dysmenorrhea that does not respond to a cyclic pill regimen. Fertil Steril 2003;80(3):560–3.

32. Zorbas KA, Economopoulos KP, Vlahos NF. Continuous versus cyclic oral contraceptives for the treatment of endometriosis: a systematic review. Arch Gynecol Obstet 2015;292(1):37–43.

33. Coffee AL, Sulak PJ, Kuehl TJ. Long-term assessment of symptomatology and satisfaction of an extended oral contraceptive regimen. Contraception 2007; 75(6):444–9.

34. Division of Reproductive Health, National Center for Chronic Disease Prevention and Health Promotion, Centers for Disease Control and Prevention (CDC). U.S. Selected Practice Recommendations for Contraceptive Use, 2013: adapted from the World Health Organization selected practice recommendations for contraceptive use, 2nd edition. MMWR Recomm Rep 2013;62(RR–05):1–60.

35. Sulak PJ, Kuehl TJ, Coffee A, et al. Prospective analysis of occurrence and management of breakthrough bleeding during an extended oral contraceptive regimen. Am J Obstet Gynecol 2006;195(4):935–41.

36. Jensen JT, Garie SG, Trummer D, et al. Bleeding profile of a flexible extended regimen of ethinylestradiol/drospirenone in US women: an open-label, three-arm, active-controlled, multicenter study. Contraception 2012;86(2):110–8.

37. Klipping C, Duijkers I, Fortier MP, et al. Long-term tolerability of ethinylestradiol 20 mug/drospirenone 3 mg in a flexible extended regimen: results from a randomised, controlled, multicentre study. J Fam Plann Reprod Health Care 2012; 38(2):84–93.

38. Guazzelli CA, Barreiros FA, Barbosa R, et al. Extended regimens of the vaginal contraceptive ring: cycle control. Contraception 2009;80(5):430–5.

39. Sulak PJ, Smith V, Coffee A, et al. Frequency and management of breakthrough bleeding with continuous use of the transvaginal contraceptive ring: a randomized controlled trial. Obstet Gynecol 2008;112(3):563–71.

40. Stewart FH, Kaunitz AM, Laguardia KD, et al. Extended use of transdermal norelgestromin/ethinyl estradiol: a randomized trial. Obstet Gynecol 2005;105(6): 1389–96.
41. van den Heuvel MW, van Bragt AJ, Alnabawy AK, et al. Comparison of ethinylestradiol pharmacokinetics in three hormonal contraceptive formulations: the vaginal ring, the transdermal patch and an oral contraceptive. Contraception 2005;72(3): 168–74.
42. Seval DL, Buckley T, Kuehl TJ, et al. Attitudes and prescribing patterns of extended-cycle oral contraceptives. Contraception 2011;84(1):71–5.

Does the Progestogen Used in Combined Hormonal Contraception Affect Venous Thrombosis Risk?

 CrossMark

Leo Han, MD*, Jeffrey T. Jensen, MD, MPH

KEYWORDS

- Progestin • Progestogen • Venous thromboembolism • Oral contraceptive
- Drospirenone

KEY POINTS

- All combined oral contraceptive pills carry a small, but increased risk for venous thromboembolism (VTE).
- Existing studies rely on observational data to estimate the risk for VTE of different progestogen subtypes.
- These studies vary in their ability to account for preexisting risk factors, confounders, and cohort-related effects.
- Despite heterogeneity in study results regarding the safety of different progestogens, the risk of VTE overall with combined oral contraceptives remains very low compared with pregnancy.
- The decision to prescribe a pill should be based on the unique risk factors and medical history of the individual woman.

INTRODUCTION

Almost 60 years after the pill first became available for contraception, more than a quarter of US women choose combined hormonal contraception (CHC) for birth control.[1] Over the years, the pill has undergone substantial modifications in chemistry, formulations, and dosing regimens, and transdermal patches and vaginal rings have been introduced. As a result, there is now a variety of combined hormonal methods to choose from. These different formulations contain both objectively demonstrated and theoretic differences in side effects and noncontraceptive benefits. Despite the

Disclosure: See last page of the article.
Department of Obstetrics and Gynecology, Oregon Health & Science University, 3181 SW Sam Jackson Park Road, Portland, OR 97239, USA
* Corresponding author. Department of Obstetrics and Gynecology, Oregon Health & Science University, 3181 SW Sam Jackson Park Road, Mailcode: L466, Portland, OR 97239.
E-mail address: hanl@ohsu.edu

Obstet Gynecol Clin N Am 42 (2015) 683–698
http://dx.doi.org/10.1016/j.ogc.2015.07.007
0889-8545/15/$ – see front matter © 2015 Elsevier Inc. All rights reserved.

obgyn.theclinics.com

options, the basic formula for CHC remains the same: an estrogen coupled with a synthetic progestogen. Consequently, the most important risk of CHC has also remained the same: venous thromboembolism (VTE).

VTE is a life-threatening condition. Two-thirds manifest as deep vein thrombosis (DVT), whereas another third present as pulmonary embolism (PE). Mortality and morbidity for these conditions are serious.[2] Studies estimate that 20% to 25% of all PE cases present as sudden death.[3] Moreover, recurrent thromboembolism, chronic venous insufficiency, and pulmonary hypertension are important nonfatal sequelae of these diseases.[4] Even in the most benign scenarios of simple, detected VTE, treatment requires a course of anticoagulation therapy that affects patient quality of life and confers risk from adverse bleeding scenarios.[5]

VTE was recognized almost immediately as a serious risk of combined oral contraceptive (COC) use. Once estrogen was identified as the culpable hormone, pharmaceutical companies scaled back the estrogen dose from what now seems like a massive load of 150 μg of mestranol per pill to modern levels of 10 to 35 μg of ethinyl estradiol (EE). As predicted, reducing estrogen doses decreased VTE risks without sacrificing efficacy. Clinicians now accept that the risk of VTE is about 2-fold higher in COC users on a background rate of about 5 to 10 per 10,000 woman-years in healthy nonpregnant women.[6] CHCs also increase the risk of arterial thromboembolism (ATE).[7] Although ATE events such as myocardial infarction (MI) and stroke are extremely rare in reproductive-aged women, the consequences are severe. However, in healthy, nonsmoking women, less than 35 years old, using low-dose (eg, <50 μg of EE) pills, the increase in risk is negligible.[8,9] Furthermore, although age, smoking, hypertension, and to a lesser extent migraine headache with aura have been reported to modify the risk of ATE[8] associated with CHC use, the type of progestogen in a formulation has not been implicated as an additional risk factor.[7] In contrast, considerable scientific debate continues regarding whether the type of progestogen used in a combined method modifies VTE risk.[10]

Because all but the most recently introduced COCs use the same synthetic estrogen, EE, the progestogen used differentiates most formulations. New progestogens were developed to address side effects related to androgenic properties of the 19-nortestosterone derivative progestogens norethindrone and levonorgestrel (LNG). This steady evolution of less androgenic progestogens led to grouping formulations into generations so that pills of similar characteristics could be discussed together. Although this classification system does not provide a true representation of structural chemistry, a body of literature had adopted the convention. However, regulatory approval of these new formulations as contraceptives did not require proof of additional health benefit or tolerability compared with existing low-dose formulations. Therefore, controversy developed because these newer progestogens were linked to an increased risk of VTE in some epidemiologic studies.[11–15]

For more than 2 decades, this controversy has persisted. Because VTE is an uncommon to rare event, phase 3 premarketing studies are underpowered to evaluate these outcomes, and are typically not conducted using an active comparator. Although case-control and database studies can provide useful insights on rare events, inherent limitations of these designs prevent ascertainment of key confounders.[10] This article examines the complex problems that obscure this debate, and highlight the merits and shortcomings of the most important and recent research contributions.

TYPES OF PROGESTOGENS

In addition to androgenicity, progestogens differ in several significant ways, including bioavailability, potency, and metabolism.[16] Individual variation in metabolism may magnify these differences, explaining why the same progestogen may have different side effects in different users.

Table 1 categorizes progestins into their respective generations. The use of the term generation is misleading, because the assignment is based not only on the derivative molecules but also on the chronologic release of the drug to market. An alternative classification system grounded in structural and biological function has been detailed by Stanczyk and colleagues.[17] This system groups progestogens according to their steroid scaffold relationship to progesterone or testosterone, and further subdivides compounds based on key substitutions to the base molecule (**Fig. 1**; see **Table 1**).[17] Progestogens structurally related to progesterone are classified as pregnanes or 19-norpregnanes based on the presence or absence of a methyl group at carbon (C)-10, and subdivided based on acetylation at C-17. Medroxyprogesterone acetate is an example of a progesterone derivative used in contraception.

The most commonly used contraceptive progestogens are derivatives of testosterone; removal of the C-19 methyl group yields the 19-nortestosterone scaffold used by all of these compounds except drospirenone (DRSP). Testosterone-derived progestogens can be further divided into those that are ethinylated (ethinyl group at

Table 1
Classification of progestogens

Progestin Generation	Parent Structure	Metabolite Family	Progestogens	Common Products
First	Testosterone (ethinylated at carbon 17)	Estrane	Norethynodrel, norethindrone, norethindrone acetate, ethynodiol diacetate	Loestrin, Ortho-Novum
Not classified	Progesterone (methylated at carbon 10)	Pregnane	Medroxyprogesterone acetate Megestrol acetate	Depo-Provera, Megace
	Progesterone (no methyl group at carbon 10)	Norpregnane	Nomegestrol acetate Nesterone	Zoely[a]
Second	Testosterone (ethinylated at carbon 13)	Gonane	Norgestrel, LNG	Mirena IUS, Lo-Ovral, Alesse, Seasonale
Third	Testosterone (ethinylated at carbon 13)	Gonane	Desogestrel, norgestimate, gestodene, etonogestrel	Ortho-Cyclen, Mircette, Femodene, Nexplanon, NuvaRing
Fourth	Testosterone (no ethinyl group at carbon 17)	Nonethinylated estrane	Drospirenone, dienogest	Yasmine, Yaz, Jeanine Natazia Qlaira

Abbreviation: IUS, intrauterine system.

[a] Not available in the United States.

Data from Stanczyk FZ, Hapgood JP, Winer S, et al. Progestogens used in postmenopausal hormone therapy: differences in their pharmacological properties, intracellular actions, and clinical effects. Endocr Rev 2013;34(2):171–208; and Hatcher RA, Trussell J, Nelson AL. Contraceptive Technology. Ardent Media; 2008.

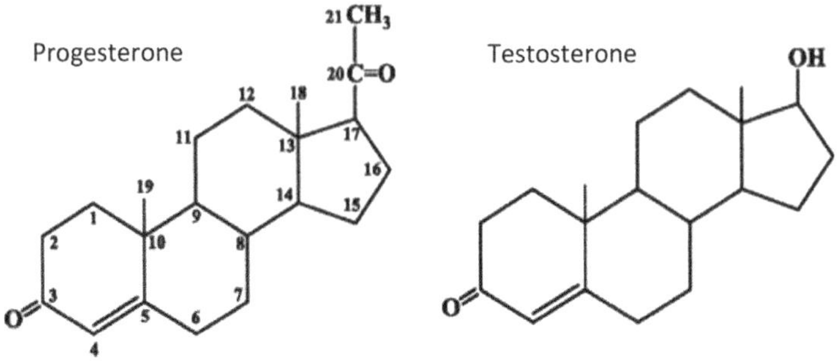

Fig. 1. Chemical structures of progesterone and testosterone with carbon numbering conventions.

C-17) or nonethinylated. The ethinylated groups include the norethindrone family of estranes as well as the LNG family of gonanes. Addition of an ethyl group at C-13 differentiates the gonanes from estranes. In the nonethinylated family, DRSP and dienogest are the most important molecules. DRSP is derived from an androstane scaffold and structurally related to spironolactone with a carbolactone group at C-17; this yields both antimineralocorticoid and antiandrogenic properties. Dienogest, a 19-nor-testosterone derivative, has a cyano group at C-17 and also possesses antiandrogenic properties. Although this categorization system makes good scientific sense, VTE epidemiologic studies heavily favor the use of the traditional generation designations.

Because of long-standing and widespread use, LNG or second-generation progestogens have emerged as the reference group for most epidemiologic studies of CHC safety. LNG has been widely used in CHC since the 1980s and is also found in several progestogen-only contraceptives including the LNG intrauterine system, contraceptive implants, and the LNG emergency birth control pill. Given its long, well-characterized history of safety and efficacy, studies usually report measures of association of newer methods relative to the VTE rates of pills containing LNG.

PHYSIOLOGY OF COMBINED ORAL CONTRACEPTIVE USE AND VENOUS THROMBOEMBOLISM

The increased risk of VTE arises from the changes that occur in the coagulation cascade brought on by estrogen. This estrogen effect represents an evolutionary adaptation of female mammals to the risk of hemorrhage that occurs with pregnancy. Estrogen leads to an increase in levels of thrombogenic clotting factors (factor I II, VII, VIII, X) as well as a decrease in levels of clotting inhibitors (tissue plasminogen activator, antiplasmin, protein S) **(Fig. 2)** that shifts the balance to favor clot formation. Several studies have shown that the type of progestogen used in a CHC influences the magnitude of the estrogen-induced changes in these various hemostatic biomarkers.[18–20] Although the biological mechanism of this progestogen effect has not been elucidated, it seems to be through modification of the estrogen response rather than a direct effect, because progestogen-only contraception does not increase VTE risk.[21] Complex interactions between estrogen, progestogen, and androgen signaling influence liver metabolism. Estrogens activate hepatic globulin synthesis. The high levels of estrogens seen by the liver following oral dosing are supraphysiologic. Although estradiol is converted to less potent estriol and estrone following the first pass, synthetic EE is more potent and also activates the liver during recirculation of

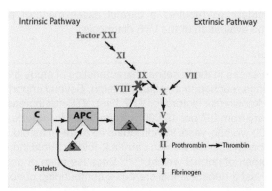

Fig. 2. The simplified coagulation cascade. Activated protein C (APC) exerts an anticoagulant effect primarily through inhibition of factor V. Protein S is required for this interaction. C, protein C. (*From* Jensen JT, Burke AE, Barnhart KT, et al. Effects of switching from oral to transdermal or transvaginal contraception on markers of thrombosis. Contraception 2008;78(6):456; with permission.)

active metabolites. These effects explain why EE increases clot risk even with transdermal or vaginal administration.[22,23]

Because many studies have shown trends toward higher levels of thrombogenic factors and suppression of thrombolytic factors in third-generation progestins compared with second-generation pills,[18–20] many experts think that the androgenic properties of a progestogen modify the estrogen effect on clotting factors. One important mediator measured in several studies is activated protein C (APC) resistance; this seems to be increased with use of third-generation compared with second-generation progestogens. APC results from the binding of protein S to protein C. Estrogens decrease levels of both of these anticoagulant factors.[24] APC acts as an anticoagulant because it terminates the clotting cascade by cleaving activated factor V and VIII.[18,20] Because APC resistance is the mechanism through which factor V Leiden mutants become hypercoagulable, there is a temptation to equate biological plausibility with true risk. However, APC resistance has never been prospectively validated as a surrogate marker for VTE.[25]

Other studies have proposed the use of sex hormone–binding globulin (SHBG) as a surrogate marker of clot risk.[26] SHBG, much like thyroid-binding globulin, is a large glycoprotein that is involved in sex hormone transport in the circulation. SHBG secretion seems to be hormonally regulated. Estrogen levels in pregnancy increase SHBG levels almost 10-fold and oral estrogens or EE by any route also result in dose-dependent increases. Similar to APC resistance, the increase in SHBG level is lower with androgenic progestogens like LNG than with less androgenic molecules like desogestrel or DRSP. However, like APC resistance, the suggestion that SHBG can serve as marker for relative estrogenicity, and in turn VTE risk, has never been validated. To date, no surrogate marker for VTE risk has been identified.[25]

BACKGROUND RISKS

Much of the criticism of early epidemiologic studies linking newer progestins to an increase in VTE risk has been a failure to address for 1 or more of the many risk factors that affect clot formation. How a study accounts and adjusts for confounding variables affect the association of progestogen type and VTE risk. Because no randomized trials exist to evaluate the differential effects of progestogens in CHC, evaluation of the validity of study outcomes requires a careful assessment of potential baseline confounders and the evaluation of the VTE diagnosis.

Confounding Factors

Unrecognized differences in the baseline characteristics of study groups threaten the validity of conclusions reached in any study design. Several important demographic characteristics are known risk factors for VTE. First, VTE risk increases with age; incidence estimates vary from 0.7 per 10,000 woman-years in individuals 15 to 19 years old to 5.8 per 10,000 woman-years in individuals 45 to 49 years old.[27] Another important risk factor is obesity. Obese women carry a 2-fold to 3-fold increased risk of VTE compared with women of normal weight.[28–30] Because rates of obesity have rapidly increased over the last 2 decades, this creates a confounding cohort effect, because the population of women enrolled in recent studies will have higher VTE rates independent of progestogen type compared with cohorts enrolled in studies 20 years ago. Related to obesity, some recent studies have suggested that polycystic ovary syndrome (PCOS) may be an independent risk factor for VTE.[31,32] Because managing symptoms of hyperandrogenism is a major therapeutic goal of PCOS treatment, providers may preferentially prescribe low-androgen pills to these high-risk women.

Other important VTE risks include smoking, malignancy, activity, and genetics. Hereditable factors are present in more than 25% of first-time VTE.[4,6,27] The factor V Leiden mutation accounts for 30% of the DVTs in the United States and its mutations are present in white people (5.3%) at a rate more than 10 times greater than in Asian people (0.5%).[19,33] The interaction of factor V Leiden and other coagulopathies such as protein C or S deficiencies and CHC use is multiplicative; the risk of clot is increased 100-fold in factor V Leiden homozygotes using CHC.[34] The high prevalence of factor V Leiden in the white population is an important factor to keep in mind because many of the large-scale database studies are conducted in Europe.

Another effect to note is the detection bias present when VTE rates from newer studies are compared with older ones. The availability of higher quality, noninvasive technologies like Doppler ultrasonography and computed tomography angiography has greatly improved the ability to see small clots. Whether or not these are clinically relevant, the increased use of these modalities in individuals perceived to be at high risk or in more recent studies may lead to bias.[35]

Risk of Venous Thromboembolism Associated with Starting or Switching a Combined Method

Multiple studies show that the risk of VTE is higher in new users.[36–38] The increased risk associated with a new prescription is independent of other known risk factors such as age and body mass index (BMI), and is estimated to be 3 times higher in the first few months of use compared with after the first year.[36] There are conflicting explanations for these phenomena. One widely accepted explanation is that continuing users make up a cohort of survivors, or women who are inherently, but perhaps intangibly, at lower risk. With the introduction of any new drug, users who are prone to adverse outcomes experience those conditions when they first begin use.[30,39] In the case of VTE, this may include women with nonclassic coagulopathies that are not picked up on screens for common mutations such as factor V Leiden. This attrition of the susceptible is reflected in new cohorts because incoming women have unknown and untested backgrounds. However, existing cohorts are made of women who have survived and are therefore healthier users, which produces a differential selection bias that could account for some of the association seen with new pills and VTE.

One biological explanation for the new-user effect is that, when initiating COC use, there is an equilibrating period when the body adjusts to the new state of hormone-induced changes in coagulation. Support for this explanation comes from studies that suggest that women who have used COCs and then discontinue reassume an increased risk when they reinitiate the same pill.[40] However, this comparison is further confounded by time, because age and changes in health status are different and therefore baseline risk may not be the same from one episode of usage to another.

Similar to new users, pill switchers are at higher risk of clot compared with continuing users, and this effect is true whether the change is from a second-generation to a third-generation or a third-generation to a second-generation pill.[40] It is possible that new combinations lead to subtle changes in the balance of procoagulation and anticoagulation factors in the liver. Changes in coagulation markers have been identified in women switching from the pill to the transdermal patch or vaginal ring.[41] Although the exact mechanism of this effect has not been elucidated, for women who develop additional risk factors, such as advancing age, weight, or inactivity, such a switch in the balance of coagulation factors may represent a destabilizing factor leading to clot formation.

Prescribing Effect

Preferential prescribing of new CHC formulations to high-risk women cannot be ruled out as the explanation for the differential VTE risks seen between progestogen type in case-control and database studies. Newer progestogens were developed and marketed with claims of decreased androgenicity to address complaints of androgen-related side effects. Because these low-androgen progestogens also lead to an increase in high-density lipoprotein cholesterol, this likely led to preferential prescription to women at risk of cardiovascular disease. A survey of German physicians showed an increased likelihood to prescribe a third-generation pill to high-risk patients and also to refer women using third-generation pills for diagnostic work-up for DVT even if symptoms were mild or nonspecific.[42] A Dutch study found that women using other cardiovascular medications were more likely to have been prescribed third-generation than second-generation pills.[43] A large prospective European cohort study showed preferential prescription of DRSP products in obese women and in women with preexisting arrhythmia, which is another risk factor for clot formation.[37]

The inverse dose response for estrogen identified by Farmer and Lawrenson[44] provides additional convincing evidence for preferential prescription bias (**Table 2**). In contrast with an expected reduction in VTE risk with decreasing dose of EE, a consistent effect of increased risk with 20-μg (introduced later) compared with 30-μg pills was identified in the World Health Organization (WHO), Transnational, and UK General Practitioner's Database studies.[45] This biologically implausible effect suggests preferential prescription of newer pills to high-risk women.

It is important to put in context the contraceptive choices available to women in the 1980s and 90s. Intrauterine device and implant use was uncommon, making the pill the most recommended contraceptive option, even in women with relative cardiovascular risk factors. It is not surprising that providers responded positively to the introduction of new COC formulations with beneficial effects on lipids.

THIRD-GENERATION AND FOURTH-GENERATION PROGESTINS: HISTORY OF THE CONTROVERSY

Whether VTE rates in users of third-generation and fourth-generation CHCs are increased in relation to second-generation pills remains highly controversial. Because

Table 2
Inverse dose-response relationships with dose of estrogen with desogestrel and cyproterone

Study[11,12,14]	Reference	Case Patients	OR	95% CI	Case Patients	OR	95% CI
		Desogestrel + 20 μg EE			Desogestrel + 30 μg EE		
WHO	Nonusers	8	38.2	4.5–325	27	7.6	3.9–14.7
Transnational	LNG	13	2.8	1.3–6.5	32	1.5	0.9–2.5
BCDSP (Jick)	LNG	4	2.7	NA	26	1.9	NA
MediPlus UK	LNG	13	2.9	0.9–10.0	19	0.6	0.3–1.5
		Cyproterone + 35 μg EE			Cyproterone + 50 μg EE		
WHO	LNG	9	5.1	1.3–20.3	9	1.3	0.5–3.8

Abbreviations: CI, confidence interval; OR, odds ratio; WHO, World Health Organization.
From Farmer RDT, Lawrenson RA. Oral contraceptives and venous thromboembolic disease: the findings from database studies in the United Kingdom and Germany. Am J Obstet Gynecol 1998;179(3 Suppl):s84; with permission.

VTE is an uncommon to rare event, a randomized controlled trial is not practical. Although case-control and database studies have found a consistent 2-fold increase in risk with third-generation and fourth-generation progestogens compared with LNG, this same effect has not been observed in large prospective cohort studies.

The First Pill Scare

Third-generation progestogens became available in COC formulations in the 1980s and rapidly gained widespread use. By the mid-1990s several observational studies suggested an increased risk of thrombosis with these pills.[11–14] The WHO case-control study found an increased risk of VTE with desogestrel (odds ratio [OR], 2.4; 95% confidence interval [CI], 1.4–4.6) and gestodene (OR, 3.1; 95% CI, 1.6–5.9) compared with LNG.[11] The transnational case-control study, conducted concurrently with the WHO, similarly found an increased OR of 1.5 (95% CI, 1.1–2.1) in comparisons of third-generation with second-generation pills.[14]

Around the same time as these case-control studies, several large database cohort studies were also done. Database studies use national identifier numbers to link health records to prescriptions, allowing researchers to perform a retrospective cohort analysis linking exposures to outcomes. Although these types of studies allow researchers to calculate incidence rates and relative risk (RR) for rare events, the retrospective nature limits the assessment of baseline confounding variables. Two prominent examples of these studies came out of the United Kingdom with conflicting results. The first, from Jick and colleagues,[12] examining the General Practitioner's Research Database, found increased RRs with gestodene (RR, 1.8; 95% CI, 1.0–3.2) and desogestrel (RR, 1.9; 95% CI, 1.1–3.2) compared with LNG. Meanwhile, Farmer and colleagues[46] probed a similar but nonoverlapping UK database of general practices (MediPlus) and performed similar cohort and nested case-control studies. Although the initial analysis showed an increased risk with third-generation pills, subanalysis showed that age was a significant confounder. Moreover, case-control analysis done in a similar way to the Jick and colleagues[12] and WHO studies led to null results when comparing gestodene and desogestrel with LNG (OR, 0.87; 95% CI, 0.4–1.8; and OR, 0.84; 95% CI, 0.4–1.9 respectively).

The Second Pill Scare

Approximately a decade later, a second wave of epidemiologic studies reignited the debate about progestogen modification of VTE risk. Results from Lidegaard and colleagues,[15] using the Danish National Database, confirmed the findings of the first pill scare showing an increased RR of VTE with desogestrel (RR, 1.82; 95% CI, 1.49–2.22) and gestodene (RR, 1.86; 95% CI, 1.59, 2.18), and found new associations with DRSP (RR, 1.64; 95% CI, 1.27–2.1) and cyproterone acetate (RR, 1.88; 95% CI, 1.47–2.42). These results were corroborated by several large case-controls studies from the United States, United Kingdom, and the Netherlands. Jick and colleagues,[47] using a US insurance claims database, found a 2-fold increase in risk for VTE among users of DRSP products (OR, 2.3; 95% CI, 1.6–3.2). A similar increase in risk for DRSP was identified in the UK General Practice Research Database (OR, 2.7; 95% CI, 1.5–4.7).[48] Most dramatically, a Dutch case-control study found a 6.3-fold increase in risk for DRSP compared with LNG (95% CI, 2.9–13.7).[49] A study performed using a health claims database from the United States came to similar conclusions.[50]

However, consistency of effect seen in these results may reflect problems inherent in the shared methodology of these studies more than a true biological association, because confounding and bias could account for the observed differences. For example, the 2009 Lidegaard and colleagues[15] study likely underestimated the rate of VTE in the LNG arm because the follow-up period started well after the introduction of LNG products, and surveillance bias might have resulted in differential diagnosis of VTE in women using the DRSP pills.

Contraceptive Ring and Patch

Nonoral forms of CHC have also the subjects of controversy and debate. There have been concerns that the transdermal patch of 0.75 mg of EE and 6 mg of norelgestromin (activate metabolite of norgestimate, a third-generation progestin) confers an increased risk for clot given higher sustained exposure to estrogen, despite lower peak levels.[51] Similar to the research seen in the pill controversies, observational data regarding its safety are conflicting. Jick and colleagues[52–54] published several nested case-control studies showing no increased risk for VTE or ATE using data from an insurance claim database compared with pills containing norgestimate or levonorgestrel. Another group using claims data from a single carrier found a 2-fold increase in VTE risk (OR, 2.0; 95% CI, 1.2–3.3) with no increased risk for ATE-related morbidity.[55,56] Database cohort studies from Lidegaard and colleagues[57] and the US Food and Drug Administration (FDA)[58] corroborated these findings. Moreover, measurements of hemostatic variables suggest changes favoring clot formation in patch users compared with COC users.[59,60] However, no prospective studies adequate to evaluate the risk of VTE in patch users have been performed to date.

The vaginal ring releases 15 μg of EE and 120 μg of etonogestrel daily. Few studies are available regarding the vaginal ring. Lidegaard and colleagues[57] used the Danish registries to evaluate clot risk in women using nonoral hormonal methods and found an increase (RR, 1.9; 95% CI, 1.3–2.7) in vaginal ring compared with LNG pill users. However, information on confounders such as smoking, family history, BMI, and thrombophilias were not reported in this study. In 2011, in response to the controversy raised by the Danish database studies, the FDA conducted a retrospective cohort study using data from 4 geographically diverse health plans that included 835,826 women with 898,251 person-years of CHC use to evaluate the risk of thrombotic and thromboembolic events and all-cause and cardiovascular mortality for 3 newer preparations (DRSP/EE pill, norelgestromin/EE patch, and the etonogestrel/EE ring). The main result of this study was a significantly higher risk of VTE in users of the patch (RR 1.55, 1.17, 2.07) and ring (RR 1.56, 1.02, 2.37) compared with low-dose pill comparators. However, because this study relied on insurance database records, no information was available on baseline confounders.[58]

Prospective Studies

True prospective research that identify baseline confounders and follow outcomes are generally considered to provide higher quality evidence that is less prone to bias than case-control or retrospective database studies.[61] To evaluate rare adverse events like VTE, large studies are required, and the expense and complexity make this type of research less common. Several important prospective studies of VTE risk have been completed in response to phase IV safety monitoring required as a condition of regulatory approval for several contraceptive products. The most important data concerning the cardiovascular safety of oral contraceptive pills come from 2 large cohort trials conducted by Dinger and colleagues.[38] The European Active Surveillance (EURAS) study enrolled 58,674 European women initiating a new prescription for combined oral contraception, and contacted subjects every 6 months to assess safety outcomes. The prospective design allowed for collection of important risk factors for VTE such as BMI. Dinger and colleagues[38] also excluded long-time users and focused on differentiating starters from switchers. Subjects contributed 142,475 woman-years of follow-up, and loss-to-follow-up rates were impressively low (2.4%). This study reflected real-world prescribing habits; providers could prescribe any pill to their patients, because there were no prescribed exclusionary criteria. Although this study did not specifically evaluate COCs by generation, no difference was found between DRSP and LNG (hazard ratio [HR], 1.0; 95% CI, 0.6–1.8) and DRSP with other oral contraceptives (HR, 0.8; 95% CI, 0.5–1.3). The subsequent International Surveillance Study of Women Taking Oral Contraceptives (INAS-OC) followed more than 85,000 women in the United States and 6 European nations for safety outcomes, including VTE, in users of 20 μg EE/3 mg DRSP on a 24/4 regimen (24 days of pills with hormones followed by 4 days of hormone-free pills). Again, this had an impressively low lost-to-follow-up rate (3.3%) and the prospective design allowed capture of confounding baseline characteristics. Similar to EURAS, there was no increased risk of VTE seen in DRSP users compared with LNG users (HR, 0.8; 95% CI, 0.4–1.3).

In addition, a large prospective study has evaluated the etonogestrel vaginal contraceptive ring.[62–64] Dinger and colleagues,[62] using essentially the same methodology as in the EURAS and INAS-OC studies, followed 33,295 subjects for a total of 66,489 woman-years. Dinger and colleagues[62] showed no difference in the risk for VTE and ATE including an HR of 0.8 (95% CI, 0.5–1.6) for VTE in ring users compared with pill users. Although all 3 of these studies were criticized for being industry funded, regulatory authorities mandated them and their protocols and analyses were reviewed and approved by independent advisory boards.

SUMMARY

Hormonal contraception remains one of the most important contributions to women's health in the last century. The birth control pill has dramatically changed the medical, social, economic, and political fates of women around the world by reducing unintended pregnancy and childbirth. Commitment to improving these drugs and ensuring their safety strengthens the benefits women derive from contraception.

The well recognized dose-dependent effects of estrogen on coagulation are undeniable. However, the comparison of those effects with the much higher physiologic levels of estrogen seen in pregnancy is important because women take oral contraceptive pills primarily to prevent pregnancy. The risk of VTE in pregnancy and the immediate postpartum period is approximately 10 to 100 times higher than with COC use.[45] Women who experience adverse cardiovascular events on COCs would also be at high risk for those events in pregnancy. There is no convincing evidence that, by avoiding CHCs, women who wish to get pregnant one day reduce their risk of a serious thrombotic event. Moreover, beyond the discussion of the increased risk for VTE, women who report ever having used a COC have lower all-cause mortalities than never-users.[14]

The progestogen modification of this risk remains controversial. Biologically plausible mechanisms and proposed surrogate markers have not been proved. Meanwhile, the epidemiologic literature is nuanced and susceptible to bias. The ease with which slight changes in methodology can alter findings reflects the small differences that are being debated and the inherent difficulty in adjusting retrospective data. At this time, the best prospective literature does not show an increased risk with use of third-generation or fourth-generation progestogens in COCs, or with the etonogestrel ring. Moreover, these data remain available for reanalysis and reappraisal.

However, the argument that the consequences of VTE are dire should not be overlooked. VTE is often a fatal event and the significance of even 1 preventable death of a young woman cannot be dismissed. Some countries, like France, have adopted a conservative approach that an LNG product should always be used for the initial

COC prescription, followed by a switch only if intolerance develops. Because these pills are also generally available at low cost, a medical economic argument can also be made for first-line prescription of LNG pills. Whether or not the safest alternative should be the default also rests on a growing but still inadequate body of literature describing the differential benefits of different progestins. Convincing literature supporting the superiority of the newer progestogens is also lacking. However, more subtle aspects of possible tolerability may emerge in the clinician-patient consultation, so policies that restrict the prescribing privileges of clinicians should be carefully reviewed and evidence based.

Ultimately, it is the individual provider's obligation to prescribe whichever contraceptive is deemed most beneficial for the individual patient. To that end, it is important to assess women who have baseline increased risks for thrombosis. Women who have risk factors such as a personal or significant family history for VTE or a concomitant medical disease should not receive a combined product. The WHO and US Centers for Disease Control and Prevention Medical Eligibility Criteria for Contraceptive Use should be consulted to determine the best contraception for women with medical comorbidities.[65,66] For most women without baseline risk factors, the use of a combined method is safe. Clinicians should present a discussion of potential risks and benefits of existing and new products to allow women to make informed choices.

DISCLOSURE OF INTEREST

L. Han states no conflict of interest and has received no payment in the preparation of this article. J.T. Jensen has received payments for consulting from Agile Pharmaceuticals, Abbvie Pharmaceuticals, Bayer Healthcare, ContraMed, Evofem Inc, HRA Pharma, Merck Pharmaceuticals, Teva Pharmaceuticals, and the Population Council. He has also received research funding from Abbvie, Bayer, the Population Council, the National Institute of Health, and the Bill and Melinda Gates Foundation. These companies and organizations may have a commercial or financial interest in the results of this research and technology. These potential conflicts of interest have been reviewed and managed by the Oregon Health & Science University.

REFERENCES

1. Mosher WD, Jones J. Use of contraception in the United States: 1982-2008. Vital Health Stat 23 2010;(29):1–44.
2. White RH. The epidemiology of venous thromboembolism. Circulation 2003; 107(23 Suppl 1):I4–8.
3. Heit JA. The epidemiology of venous thromboembolism in the community. Arterioscler Thromb Vasc Biol 2008;28(3):370–2.
4. Beckman MG, Hooper WC, Critchley SE, et al. Venous thromboembolism. Am J Prev Med 2010;38(4):S495–501.
5. Kahn SR, Ducruet T, Lamping DL, et al. Prospective evaluation of health-related quality of life in patients with deep venous thrombosis. Arch Intern Med 2005; 165(10):1173–8.
6. Heinemann LAJ, Dinger JC. Range of published estimates of venous thromboembolism incidence in young women. Contraception 2007;75(5):328–36.
7. Lidegaard Ø, Løkkegaard E, Jensen A, et al. Thrombotic stroke and myocardial infarction with hormonal contraception. N Engl J Med 2012;366(24):2257–66.
8. Ischaemic stroke and combined oral contraceptives: results of an international, multicentre, case-control study. WHO Collaborative Study of Cardiovascular Disease and Steroid Hormone Contraception. Lancet 1996;348(9026):498–505.

9. Margolis KL, Adami H-O, Luo J, et al. A prospective study of oral contraceptive use and risk of myocardial infarction among Swedish women. Fertil Steril 2007; 88(2):310–6.

10. Bitzer J, Amy J-J, Beerthuizen R, et al. Statement on combined hormonal contraceptives containing third- or fourth-generation progestogens or cyproterone acetate, and the associated risk of thromboembolism. J Fam Plann Reprod Health Care 2013;39(3):156–9.

11. Venous thromboembolic disease and combined oral contraceptives: results of international multicentre case-control study. World Health Organization Collaborative Study of Cardiovascular Disease and Steroid Hormone Contraception. Lancet 1995;346(8990):1575–82.

12. Jick H, Jick SS, Gurewich V, et al. Risk of idiopathic cardiovascular death and nonfatal venous thromboembolism in women using oral contraceptives with differing progestagen components. Lancet 1995;346(8990):1589–93.

13. Bloemenkamp KWM, Helmerhorst FM, Rosendaal FR, et al. Enhancement by factor V Leiden mutation of risk of deep-vein thrombosis associated with oral contraceptives containing a third-generation progestagen. Lancet 1995;346(8990):1593–6.

14. Spitzer WO, Lewis MA, Heinemann LA, et al. Third generation oral contraceptives and risk of venous thromboembolic disorders: an international case-control study. Transnational Research Group on Oral Contraceptives and the Health of Young Women. BMJ 1996;312(7023):83–8.

15. Lidegaard O, Lokkegaard E, Svendsen AL, et al. Hormonal contraception and risk of venous thromboembolism: national follow-up study. BMJ 2009; 339(aug13 2):b2890.

16. Stanczyk FZ. All progestins are not created equal. Steroids 2003;68(10–13): 879–90.

17. Stanczyk FZ, Hapgood JP, Winer S, et al. Progestogens used in postmenopausal hormone therapy: differences in their pharmacological properties, intracellular actions, and clinical effects. Endocr Rev 2013;34(2):171–208.

18. Oral Contraceptive and Hemostasis Study Group. The effects of seven monophasic oral contraceptive regimens on hemostatic variables: conclusions from a large randomized multicenter study. Contraception 2003;67(3):173–85.

19. Vandenbroucke JP, Koster T, Rosendaal FR, et al. Increased risk of venous thrombosis in oral-contraceptive users who are carriers of factor V Leiden mutation. Lancet 1994;344(8935):1453–7.

20. Kemmeren JM, Algra A, Meijers JCM, et al. Effect of second- and third-generation oral contraceptives on the protein C system in the absence or presence of the factor V Leiden mutation: a randomized trial. Blood 2004;103(3):927–33.

21. Mantha S, Karp R, Raghavan V, et al. Assessing the risk of venous thromboembolic events in women taking progestin-only contraception: a meta-analysis. BMJ 2012;345(aug07 2):e4944.

22. Ansbacher R. The pharmacokinetics and efficacy of different estrogens are not equivalent. Am J Obstet Gynecol 2001;184(3):255–63.

23. Canonico M, Oger E, Plu-Bureau G, et al. Hormone therapy and venous thromboembolism among postmenopausal women: impact of the route of estrogen administration and progestogens: the ESTHER Study. Circulation 2007;115(7):840–5.

24. Tchaikovski SN, Rosing J. Mechanisms of estrogen-induced venous thromboembolism. Thromb Res 2010;126(1):5–11.

25. Stanczyk FZ, Grimes DA. Sex hormone-binding globulin: not a surrogate marker for venous thromboembolism in women using oral contraceptives. Contraception 2008;78(3):201–3.

26. Odlind V, Milsom I, Persson I, et al. Can changes in sex hormone binding globulin predict the risk of venous thromboembolism with combined oral contraceptive pills? Acta Obstet Gynecol Scand 2002;81(6):482–90.

27. Lidegaard Ø, Milsom I, Geirsson RT, et al. Hormonal contraception and venous thromboembolism. Acta Obstet Gynecol Scand 2012;91(7):769–78.

28. Edelman A, Jensen J. Obesity and hormonal contraception: safety and efficacy. Semin Reprod Med 2012;30(06):479–85.

29. Edelman A. Contraceptive considerations in obese women. Contraception 2009; 80(6):583–90.

30. Shapiro S, Dinger J. Risk of venous thromboembolism among users of oral contraceptives: a review of two recently published studies. J Fam Plann Reprod Health Care 2010;36(1):33–8.

31. Okoroh EM, Hooper WC, Atrash HK, et al. Is polycystic ovary syndrome another risk factor for venous thromboembolism? United States, 2003–2008. Am J Obstet Gynecol 2012;207(5):377.e1–8.

32. Bird ST, Hartzema AG, Brophy JM, et al. Risk of venous thromboembolism in women with polycystic ovary syndrome: a population-based matched cohort analysis. Can Med Assoc J 2013;185(2):E115–20.

33. Bloemenkamp KWM, Helmerhorst FM, Rosendaal FR, et al. Thrombophilias and gynaecology. Best Pract Res Clin Obstet Gynaecol 2003;17(3):509–28.

34. Hatcher RA, Trussell J, Nelson AL. Contraceptive technology. New York: Ardent Media; 2008.

35. Wells P, Anderson D. The diagnosis and treatment of venous thromboembolism. Hematology Am Soc Hematol Educ Program 2013;2013(1):457–63.

36. Suissa S, Blais L, Spitzer WO, et al. First-time use of newer oral contraceptives and the risk of venous thromboembolism. Contraception 1997;56(3):141–6.

37. Dinger JC, Heinemann LAJ, Kühl-Habich D. The safety of a drospirenone-containing oral contraceptive: final results from the European Active Surveillance Study on Oral Contraceptives based on 142,475 women-years of observation. Contraception 2007;75(5):344–54.

38. Dinger J, Bardenheuer K, Heinemann K. Cardiovascular and general safety of a 24-day regimen of drospirenone-containing combined oral contraceptives: final results from the International Active Surveillance Study of Women Taking Oral Contraceptives. Contraception 2014;89(4):253–63.

39. Speroff L, Darney PD. A clinical guide for contraception. Philadelphia: Lippincott Williams & Wilkins; 2010.

40. Suissa S, Spitzer WO, Rainville B, et al. Recurrent use of newer oral contraceptives and the risk of venous thromboembolism. Hum Reprod 2000;15(4): 817–21.

41. Jensen JT, Burke AE, Barnhart KT, et al. Effects of switching from oral to transdermal or transvaginal contraception on markers of thrombosis. Contraception 2008;78(6):451–8.

42. Heinemann LAJ, Lewis MA, Assmann A, et al. Could preferential prescribing and referral behaviour of physicians explain the elevated thrombosis risk found to be associated with third generation oral contraceptives? Pharmacoepidemiol Drug Saf 1996;5(5):285–94.

43. Herings R, Urquhart J, Leufkens H. Venous thromboembolism among new users of different oral contraceptives. Lancet 1999;354(9173):127–8.

44. Farmer RDT, Lawrenson RA. Oral contraceptives and venous thromboembolic disease: the findings from database studies in the United Kingdom and Germany. Am J Obstet Gynecol 1998;179(3 Supplement):s78–86.

45. Lewis MA, Heinemann LAJ, MacRae KD, et al. The increased risk of venous thromboembolism and the use of third generation progestagens: role of bias in observational research. Contraception 1996;54(1):5–13.
46. Farmer R, Lawrenson R, Thompson C, et al. Population-based study of risk of venous thromboembolism associated with various oral contraceptives. Lancet 1997;349(9045):83–8.
47. Jick SS, Hernandez RK. Risk of non-fatal venous thromboembolism in women using oral contraceptives containing drospirenone compared with women using oral contraceptives containing levonorgestrel: case-control study using United States claims data. BMJ 2011;342(apr21 2):d2151.
48. Parkin L, Sharples K, Hernandez RK, et al. Risk of venous thromboembolism in users of oral contraceptives containing drospirenone or levonorgestrel: nested case-control study based on UK General Practice Research Database. BMJ 2011;342(apr21 2):d2139.
49. Van Hylckama Vlieg A, Helmerhorst FM, Vandenbroucke JP, et al. The venous thrombotic risk of oral contraceptives, effects of oestrogen dose and progestogen type: results of the MEGA case-control study. BMJ 2009;339(aug13 2): b2921.
50. Research C for DE and. Drug Safety and Availability - FDA drug safety communication: Updated information about the risk of blood clots in women taking birth control pills containing drospirenone. Available at: http://www.fda.gov/Drugs/DrugSafety/ucm299305.htm. Accessed March 3, 2015.
51. Van den Heuvel MW, van Bragt AJM, Alnabawy AKM, et al. Comparison of ethinylestradiol pharmacokinetics in three hormonal contraceptive formulations: the vaginal ring, the transdermal patch and an oral contraceptive. Contraception 2005;72(3):168–74.
52. Jick S, Kaye JA, Li L, et al. Further results on the risk of nonfatal venous thromboembolism in users of the contraceptive transdermal patch compared to users of oral contraceptives containing norgestimate and 35 µg of ethinyl estradiol. Contraception 2007;76(1):4–7.
53. Jick SS, Hagberg KW, Hernandez RK, et al. Postmarketing study of ORTHO EVRA® and levonorgestrel oral contraceptives containing hormonal contraceptives with 30 mcg of ethinyl estradiol in relation to nonfatal venous thromboembolism. Contraception 2010;81(1):16–21.
54. Jick SS, Kaye JA, Russmann S, et al. Risk of nonfatal venous thromboembolism in women using a contraceptive transdermal patch and oral contraceptives containing norgestimate and 35 µg of ethinyl estradiol. Contraception 2006; 73(3):223–8.
55. Dore DD, Norman H, Loughlin J, et al. Extended case-control study results on thromboembolic outcomes among transdermal contraceptive users. Contraception 2010;81(5):408–13.
56. Cole JA, Norman H, Doherty M, et al. Venous thromboembolism, myocardial infarction, and stroke among transdermal contraceptive system users. Obstet Gynecol 2007;109(2, Part 1):339–46.
57. Lidegaard Ø, Nielsen LH, Skovlund CW, et al. Venous thrombosis in users of non-oral hormonal contraception: follow-up study, Denmark 2001-10. BMJ 2012;344: e2990.
58. US Food and Drug Administration, Office of Surveillance and Epidemiology. Combined hormonal contraceptives (CHCs) and the risk of cardiovascular disease endpoints. Available at: www.fda.gov/downloads/Drugs/DrugSafety/UCM277384.pdf. Accessed May 21, 2015.

59. Johnson JV, Lowell J, Badger GJ, et al. Effects of oral and transdermal hormonal contraception on vascular risk markers: a randomized controlled trial. Obstet Gynecol 2008;111(2 Pt 1):278–84.

60. White T, Ozel B, Jain JK, et al. Effects of transdermal and oral contraceptives on estrogen-sensitive hepatic proteins. Contraception 2006;74(4):293–6.

61. Schulz KF, Grimes DA. The Lancet handbook of essential concepts in clinical research. Philadelphia: Elsevier; 2006.

62. Dinger J, Möhner S, Heinemann K. Cardiovascular risk associated with the use of an etonogestrel-containing vaginal ring. Obstet Gynecol 2013;122(4):800–8.

63. Reid RL, Westhoff C, Mansour D, et al. Oral Contraceptives and venous thromboembolism consensus opinion from an International Workshop held in Berlin, Germany in December 2009. J Fam Plann Reprod Health Care 2010;36(3):117–22.

64. Vessey M, Yeates D, Flynn S. Factors affecting mortality in a large cohort study with special reference to oral contraceptive use. Contraception 2010;82(3): 221–9.

65. WHO. Medical eligibility criteria for contraceptive use. WHO. Available at: http://www.who.int/reproductivehealth/publications/family_planning/9789241563888/en/. Accessed May 18, 2015.

66. CDC - United States medical eligibility criteria (USMEC) for contraceptive use - reproductive health. Available at: http://www.cdc.gov/reproductivehealth/unintendedpregnancy/usmec.htm. Accessed July 28, 2014.

Emergency Contraception
Do Your Patients Have a Plan B?

Holly Bullock, MD, MPH*, Jennifer Salcedo, MD, MPH, MPP

KEYWORDS

- Emergency contraception • Copper intrauterine device • Ulipristal acetate
- Levonorgestrel • Access

KEY POINTS

- Emergency contraception (EC) is used to decrease the risk of pregnancy after unprotected intercourse, inadequately protected intercourse, or sexual assault.
- The copper intrauterine device (Cu-IUD) is the most effective method of EC and should be placed within 5 days of intercourse, or within 5 days of estimated ovulation.
- Ulipristal acetate (UPA) is the most effective oral method of EC approved in the United States. It requires a prescription and should be taken as soon as possible within 120 hours of intercourse.
- Levonorgestrel emergency contraceptive pills (ECPs) should be taken as soon as possible after intercourse and maintain some efficacy up to 120 hours. A branded single-dose levonorgestrel ECP is available over-the-counter without age restrictions.
- Women are at increased risk of ECP failure if they are overweight, have unprotected intercourse during the most fertile time of their cycle, or have multiple episodes of unprotected intercourse during one cycle.

INTRODUCTION

Emergency contraception (EC) is a drug or device used following unprotected or inadequately protected intercourse to reduce risk of pregnancy. Although overall contraceptive use in the United States is high, with 99% of sexually active women reporting ever using a method in their lifetime, the most popular methods carry a significant risk of failure during typical use.[1–3] According to the Survey of Family Growth, 49.5 million women have used male condoms, 43.8 million oral contraceptive pills, and 31.3 million withdrawal.[4] The use of emergency contraceptive pills (ECPs) is also on

Disclosure Statement: The authors have nothing to disclose.
Department of Obstetrics, Gynecology, and Women's Health, University of Hawaii John A. Burns School of Medicine, 1319 Punahou Street, Suite 824, Honolulu, HI 96826, USA
* Corresponding author.
E-mail address: bullockh@hawaii.edu

the rise, with ever use increasing from 4% to 10% between 2002 and 2008.[4] Given that more than half of women experiencing unintended pregnancy report attempting contraception when they conceived, experts recommend that all women using contraception should be provided with detailed counseling on EC use.[1,5] In the United States, current EC options include the copper intrauterine device (Cu-IUD), ulipristal acetate (UPA), levonorgestrel-containing ECP (LNG-ECP), and the Yuzpe method of combined oral contraceptives (COCs). **Figs. 1** and **2** visually compare efficacy of the most effective methods and timing of administration.

Evidence is inconsistent as to whether increased access to EC decreases use of regular contraception or increases other sexual risk-taking behavior. In a study of 1490 women aged 24 to 24 not using long-acting reversible contraception, Raymond and Weaver[6] found that those randomized to advanced provision of ECPs exhibited an increased likelihood of unprotected and underprotected sex, compared with those who had to present in-person for care when ECPs were needed. In a subanalysis of that same cohort, Weaver and colleagues[7] found that women randomized to receive increased access to EC were more likely to substitute EC for their "typical" contraceptive. This was particularly true of those relying on condoms. In contrast, in a randomized control trial across four California clinics, Raine and colleagues[8] demonstrated that advanced provision of ECPs did not increase rates of unprotected sex or sexually transmitted infections (STIs). A 2007 Cochrane Review on advance provision of ECPs also reported no difference in rates of STIs, frequency of unprotected coitus, or changes in contraceptive methods across the eight trials that met inclusion criteria.

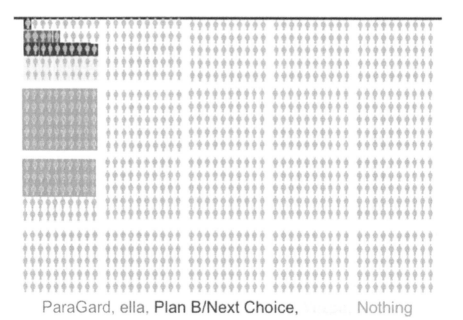

ParaGard, ella, Plan B/Next Choice, Nothing

Fig. 1. Pregnancies per 1000 women after unprotected intercourse using various methods of EC compared with no EC. *Blue*: Cu-IUD as EC, less than 1 in 1000 pregnancies. *Red*: UPA, with 5 in 1000 pregnancies. *Pink*: LNG-ECP, with 10 in 1000 pregnancies. *Yellow*: the Yuzpe regimen of COC, with 20 in 1000 pregnancies. *Green*: no method of EC used, 80 in 1000 pregnancies. (*From* Trussell J. Update on emergency contraception, Slide #18 [PowerPoint Slide]. 6/18/2014. Association of Reproductive Health Professionals. Available at: www.arhp.org/core. Accessed May 14, 2015.)

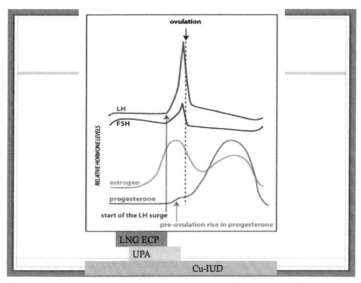

Fig. 2. Relative hormone levels preceding ovulation vis à vis timing of EC. LNG-ECP (*brown bar*) is effective in delaying ovulation 76% to 89% when taken before the LH surge (*red*).[55] UPA (*green bar*), the progesterone modulator, is effective in delaying ovulation 100% when taken before the LH surge as the progesterone levels are rising; rates of ovulation delay are 79% if taken before the LH peak.[54,55] The Cu-IUD (*pink bar*) is nearly 100% effective in preventing pregnancy when used up to 5 days after ovulation, primarily through altering motility and fertilizing ability of sperm. It can be used at any point during the cycle.[22] FSH, follicle-stimulating hormone; LH, luteinizing hormone. (*Adapted from* Hormonal contraception. Available at: http://courses.washington.edu/conj/bess/contraception/contraception.htm. Accessed May 14, 2015; and *Data from* Refs.[22,54,55])

Of note, advance provision did not reduce pregnancy rates when compared with standard access, but did increase the use of EC.[9]

These findings indicate that access to EC alone is not a panacea. Rather, it should be the starting point for a discussion on EC, other contraceptive options highlighting long-acting reversible contraception, and the importance of dual method use with condoms to prevent STIs.

PREGNANCY RISK

The risk of pregnancy following a single act of intercourse is estimated to be 4% to 6% overall, increasing to 30% during the most fertile time of the cycle.[10,11] Generally, the fertile period of the menstrual cycle is considered to last 6 days, ending on the day of ovulation, after which the ova has 24 hours to be fertilized before disintegration.[11–13] Spermatozoa in the female reproductive tract retain their ability to fertilize an ovum for 5 to 6 days.[14,15] Additionally, the timing of ovulation can vary between cycles, taking place between Days 10 and 21 of the cycle, but occurring most frequently between Days 13 to 16.[16] Given the uncertainty of ovulation timing and the prolonged viability of sperm, women should be encouraged to use EC when inadequately protected intercourse occurs at any point in the menstrual cycle (**Table 1**). New data indicate that women are more likely to engage in unprotected sex closer to ovulation, increasing risk of pregnancy.[17] A single act of intercourse takes place in the fertile window of a woman's cycle one out of four times.[17]

Table 1
Indications for emergency contraceptive use

Method of Contraception	Indication
None	Always indicated[a]
Lactation amenorrhea method[b]	Criteria for method no longer met and no use of additional methods
Hormonal methods	
Progestin-only contraceptive pills	Delay since last pill >27 h Vomiting, diarrhea for >48 h Delay in starting new pill pack No backup method first 2 d of method
Combined oral contraceptive pills	Two or more missed pills Delay in starting new pill pack by >48 h Vomiting and diarrhea for >48 h No backup method first 7 d of method
Patch	Leaving the patch on for >9 d Delay in applying new patch >48 h No backup method first 7 d of method
Ring	Leaving the ring in for >35 d Failure to reinsert ring >48 h No backup method first 7 d of method
Depot medroxyprogesterone acetate injection	Interval between injections >15 wk No backup method first 7 d of method
Barrier methods	
Male condom	Slippage, leakage, breakage
Female condom	Incorrect insertion, dislodgement
Diaphragm, cervical cap	Incorrect insertion, dislodgement
Spermicide	Incorrect insertion, failure to melt
Withdrawal	Incorrect or uncertain usage
Long-acting reversible methods	
Copper IUD	Concern for device expulsion Device beyond duration of efficacy
LNG IUD	Concern for device expulsion Device beyond duration of efficacy No backup method first 7 d of method
Progestin implant	Device beyond duration of efficacy No backup method first 7 d of method

[a] EC use is always indicated for unprotected sex and after sexual assault.
[b] Criteria for lactation amenorrhea method include: (1) infant is <6 months of age; (2) fully breast-feeding every 4 hours or less during the day, up to every 6 hours at night or (3) nearly fully breast-feeding every 4 hours or less during the day, up to every 6 hours at night, with 5% to 15% of feeds supplementation by other means; and (4) no resumption of menses postpartum.
From Hatcher R, Trussell J, Nelson AL, et al, editors. Contraceptive technology. 20th revised edition. New York: Ardent Media; 2011; with permission.

Effective use of EC requires women to realize they are at risk for pregnancy and take action. However, up to 40% of women in the United States are unaware of when during the cycle they are the most fertile.[18,19] Similarly, many women with access to ECPs fail to use the medication when indicated.[20] In a California-based trial, nearly half of women who received an advanced supply of ECPs did not use them after unprotected sex. In another trial conducted in Nevada and North Carolina, one-third of participants in an EC advance provision group had unprotected sex at least once during the year-long study period without using ECP.[8,20–22]

THE MOST EFFECTIVE EMERGENCY CONTRACEPTION: THE COPPER INTRAUTERINE DEVICE

The Cu-IUD was first described as a method of EC in 1976.[23] In a meta-analysis of 42 published articles including more than 7000 postcoital insertions of the Cu-IUD, only 10 failures were reported, yielding a pregnancy rate of 0.1%.[22,24,25] To prevent pregnancy, the Cu-IUD should be placed within 5 days of unprotected sex or within 5 days of predicted ovulation in a woman with regular menstrual cycles.[22,26,27] In one trial of 1963 women receiving the Cu-IUD as EC, the effectiveness was 100% in preventing pregnancy.[23] In this study, only 5.6% of users discontinued the method by 12 months, indicating many women will continue to use this highly effective method.[23] Similarly, in their trial of 1013 women receiving the IUD for EC, Zhou and Xiao[28] found that 96% of parous women and 80% of nulliparous women maintained the device for ongoing contraception.

Outside of research studies clinicians often do not recommend the Cu-IUD as a method of EC. In a survey of California health care providers participating in the Family Planning, Access, Care, and Treatment (FamilyPACT) program, 85% had never recommended the Cu-IUD for EC, and only 1.7% had recommended it 10 or more times.[29] Clinicians who routinely counseled patients on IUDs for regular contraception were no more likely to recommend it as a method of EC than their colleagues who did not routinely provide IUDs.[29]

Mechanism of Action

Cu-IUDs work primarily by impairing the motility, viability, and acrosomal reaction of sperm.[30–37] Copper may also have an ovicidal effect and may destroy a fertilized ovum, and recruit leukocytes, alter cell metabolism, and create a toxic environment preventing implantation.[31,38–41]

Safety

Almost all women can safely use a Cu-IUD. Limited contraindications include suspicion of current pregnancy, some cancers of the genital tract, Wilson disease, current purulent cervicitis, untreated chlamydia or gonorrhea, recent uterine infection, and uterine malformations that preclude insertion.[1,42,43] Fibroids are not a contraindication to insertion.[43] In asymptomatic women, IUD insertion should not be postponed until results of STI testing are available. Instead, STI screening may be performed at the time of insertion, if indicated.[27] Small risks of Cu-IUD insertion include perforation (approximately 1 in 1000) and increased risk of infection during the first 3 weeks (from 1.4 to 9.7 infections per 1000 woman-years).[1,44–47] In the very rare event that pregnancy occurs despite use of the Cu-IUD for EC, the device should be removed as soon as possible if technically feasible. Women with retained IUD during pregnancy are at elevated risk of spontaneous abortion, preterm delivery, septic abortion, and chorioamnionitis. If the IUD is removed, risks decrease, but do not return to baseline levels.[30,31,48]

Side Effects

After insertion, some women experience intermenstrual bleeding, increased dysmenorrhea, and modest increases in menstrual bleeding volume. However, many notice diminishing symptoms over time if the IUD is continued.[44,49] Even in women with iron deficiency anemia, the increase in menstrual bleeding associated with Cu-IUD use is less likely to deplete iron stores than a pregnancy carried to term. Use up to 5 years does not clinically impact iron stores.[43] Up to 5% of users have an expulsion and need to have the device replaced or transition to another method.[42,44,47,49,50]

DEDICATED ORAL FORMS OF EMERGENCY CONTRACEPTION
Ulipristal Acetate

UPA is a second-generation selective progesterone receptor modulator taken as a one-time 30-mg dose. UPA was first approved by European Medicines Agency in May 2009 and approved by the US Food and Drug Administration (FDA) in June 2010.[30] UPA requires a prescription. According to package instructions, it must be taken within 120 hours of unprotected intercourse.[43]

Efficacy
In a noninferiority trial of ECP use within 72 hours of unprotected intercourse, UPA users experienced an 85% reduction in expected pregnancies compared with a 69% reduction with LNG-ECPs.[51] Similarly, a randomized noninferiority trial by Glasier and colleagues[52] demonstrated that UPA resulted in 66% fewer pregnancies than LNG at 24 hours, and 50% fewer pregnancies at 120 hours. Although working via a similar mechanism of action, UPA is superior to LNG in delaying ovulation. As body mass index (BMI) increases, LNG and UPA both seem to exhibit decreased efficacy. In a study by Glasier and colleagues,[10] LNG-ECPs became ineffective in women with a BMI greater than 26 kg/m^2, whereas UPA was found to remain effective up to BMI of approximately 35 kg/m^2. However, further research is needed to elucidate the association between body weight and BMI and the effectiveness of EC.[53]

Mechanism of action
UPA works by delaying ovulation. When administered before the luteinizing hormone (LH) surge, it inhibits 100% of follicular rupture.[54] If women are treated after the onset of the LH surge but before its peak, 79% still have prevention of follicular rupture within 5 days. In contrast, only 8% of women have delayed follicular rupture if UPA is taken after the LH peak.[54,55] When taken as a 30-mg dose, UPA does not seem to have post-fertilization effects. Dose-dependent effects of progesterone receptor modulators on the endometrium include thinning and delay in maturation. However, the endometrial effects of a single 30-mg dose are similar to placebo.[30,56]

Safety
No deaths or serious complications have been reported in association with UPA.[1,57] Of pregnancies exposed to UPA, no increase in spontaneous abortion, poor pregnancy outcomes, or teratogenicity have been reported.[24,58] When used as an EC, UPA does not have any medical contraindications.[59]

The most commonly reported side effects of UPA from postmarketing data include gastrointestinal symptoms (nausea, abdominal pain, and vomiting), neurologic symptoms (headache and dizziness), and reproductive complaints (heavy vaginal bleeding, delay of menstruation, and breast tenderness).[60] UPA and LNG have similar rates of reported side effects, such as headache, dysmenorrhea, nausea, and menstrual disturbances.[1,52]

Based on the lack of data on the level of UPA excretion in breast milk, UPA packaging does not recommend use by breastfeeding women.[59,61] Mifepristone, an anti-progestin used in US medical abortion regimens, reaches concentrations in breast milk of only 1.5% maternal serum concentrations.[62] Given that UPA is similarly lipophilic, some experts recommend cessation of breastfeeding for 36 hours after UPA use when it is taken by breastfeeding women.[31]

Levonorgestrel-Containing Emergency Contraceptive Pill

Plan B One-Step is a single 1.5-mg LNG-ECP that received FDA approval in 2009 for over-the-counter purchase, and is now available without age restrictions.[1,22] Women are recommended to take the entire 1.5-mg dose at once as soon as possible after intercourse rather than as two doses separated by 12 hours. According to the manufacturer's instructions, it should be taken within 72 hours of unprotected intercourse. However, efficacy has been demonstrated up to 120 hours after unprotected intercourse.[63,64] Generic forms of the 1.5-mg LNG-ECPs can be obtained with a prescription.[22]

Efficacy

The reported efficacy of LNG-ECPs varies widely. In trials conducted by the World Health Organization, reduction in anticipated pregnancies was noted to be 95%, 85%, and 58% when LNG-ECPs were used within 24 hours, 25 to 48 hours, and 49 to 72 hours, respectively.[52,65] When LNG-ECPs have been compared with the Yuzpe method, they prevented at least 49% of expected pregnancies.[13] An additional eight studies, for a combined total of more than 9500 women, found the effectiveness of LNG to range from 59% to 94%.[21,65–70]

Mechanism of action

LNG as an EC has no effects on endometrial morphology or markers of receptivity, and has no impact on embryo viability or attachment.[31] LNG-ECPs work by delaying follicular development after the selection of the dominant follicle, before the LH surge. When LNG-ECPs were taken before the LH surge, delay of ovulation occurred in 79% to 86% of women compared with 13% to 56% of women who took placebo.[55]

The ability of LNG-ECP to inhibit or delay ovulation depends on follicle size. When dominant follicles measured between 12 to 17 mm, delay in ovulation occurred in 93% of cycles treated with LNG-ECP.[55] When dominant follicles were more than 18 mm in diameter, or when LH had started to rise, ovulation was not inhibited.[55] The effect of LNG on follicular development is either through delay of follicular development or arrest of persistent, unruptured follicles.[55]

Safety

LNG exposure is not associated with teratogenicity or adverse pregnancy outcomes.[31,71] LNG is well tolerated and is not allergenic.[5,72,73] The Centers for Disease Control and Prevention's US Medically Eligible Criteria for Contraceptive Use recognizes no contraindications to LNG EC use.[43,63] The US Medically Eligible Criteria for Contraceptive Use also specifies that women with cardiovascular disease, migraines, liver disease, history of previous ectopic pregnancy, and women who are breastfeeding may use LNG-ECPs if needed.[43] LNG is detectable in breast milk for 8 to 12 hours after ingestion but no adverse effects of progestin exposure have been noted in infants exposed to other methods of LNG-containing contraception. LNG also does not impact breastfeeding performance, with few reports of decreased volume.[63,74] Both the American Congress of Obstetricians and Gynecologists and World Health Organization agree that breastfeeding is safe for women using LNG-ECPs.[30,75]

THE YUZPE METHOD

For women with no access to other dedicated ECP products, the Yuzpe method remains an option. The Yuzpe method is less effective than LNG and UPA and has higher rates of gastrointestinal side effects.[31,52,76,77] First described in 1974, the Yuzpe method consists of two doses of COCs taken 12 hours apart. Each dose includes 100-μg ethinyl estradiol and 0.5 mg LNG. Any brand of COC may be used as long as it provides the required amount of estrogen and progestin.[76] Extensive research over the past 50 years has confirmed that the use of combined hormonal contraception during early pregnancy carries no risk to the embryo.[5,78] The FDA removed the warnings about possible teratogenic effects from the labels of COCs more than a decade ago.[5] There are no medical contraindications to the Yuzpe method. Despite the brief period of estrogen exposure, the potential benefit of pregnancy prevention outweighs the theoretic risk of venous thromboembolism and other adverse events, even for women in whom COCs are contraindicated.[22,43]

ORAL EMERGENCY CONTRACEPTION INTERACTIONS WITH OTHER MEDICATIONS

UPA does not induce or inhibit the cytochrome P-450 enzymes.[59] Consequently, no drug-drug interaction in vivo studies have been performed. UPA is metabolized primarily by CYP3A4.[59] A theoretic risk that inducers and inhibitors of this enzyme could affect the metabolism of UPA has been noted. Inducers of CYP3A4 activity, such as barbiturates, bosentan, rifampin, dexamethasone, St. John's wort, phenytoin, phenobarbital, carbamazepine, griseofulvin, and topiramate, could lower the plasma volume of UPA[31,59,75] possibly resulting in decreased effectiveness.[59,75] LNG-ECPs may also have altered efficacy from the same CYP3A4 inducers, and HIV protease inhibitors and nonnucleoside reverse-transcriptase inhibitors.[63] Although no clinical evidence of decreased efficacy caused by drug-drug interactions exists, some experts consider increasing the dose of ECPs in such circumstances.[22] Women taking these medications should still take oral EC as soon as possible after unprotected or inadequately protected intercourse, and contact their clinician to discuss possible Cu-IUD placement.

WHEN TO START CONTRACEPTION AFTER EMERGENCY CONTRACEPTION

All methods of contraception except the LNG-IUD can be started immediately following ECP use.[30] A theoretic concern exists for decreased effectiveness of progestin-containing contraceptives after use of UPA.[1,22,30,59,75] To address this potential risk the UPA manufacturer recommends a back-up barrier method with each act of coitus until the next menstrual cycle.[59]

IUD insertion in the setting of early, undiagnosed pregnancy is associated with risks of spontaneous abortion, preterm delivery, septic abortion, and chorioamnionitis.[30,31,48] Consequently, IUD insertion (outside of the Cu-IUD insertion for EC) should generally be deferred until the clinician is confident that pregnancy has been excluded. Clinicians should refer to the US Selected Practice Recommendation for Contraceptive Use on how to be reasonably certain that the woman is not pregnant.[27] Criteria include absence of pregnancy symptoms and any one of the following criteria: ≤7 days after the start of normal menses; no sexual intercourse since the start of the last normal menses; correct and consistent use of a reliable form of contraception; ≤7 days after spontaneous abortion or induced abortion; less than 4 weeks after delivery, or if patient is using the lactational amenorrhea method.[27]

INCREASING ACCESS TO EMERGENCY CONTRACEPTION

The American Congress of Obstetricians and Gynecologists recommends that EC counseling be integrated into all clinical visits for reproductive-age women, providing written information and advance prescriptions.[79] The American Academy of Pediatrics similarly recommends that all adolescents (males and females) and families of disabled adolescents should be counseled on EC as part of routine anticipatory guidance and recommends advance provision of LNG-ECPs.[80] The American Association of Family Practitioners,[81] Society of Adolescent Health and Medicine,[82] Association of Reproductive Health Professionals,[83] and the American Public Health Association[84] have all issued similar recommendations.

In 2010 more than 4 million US women used LNG-ECPs.[85] One study modeled the impact of wider availability of UPA, and found replacing those 4.17 million doses of LNG-ECP with UPA would result in 37,589 fewer unintended births in the United States annually. This amounts to an annual cost savings to Medicaid programs of $116.3 million.[86] However, limitations caused by insurance coverage,[87] lack of pharmacy availability,[1,87,88] and pharmacist misinformation[85,89] often preclude access to UPA.

Although not a cost-saving intervention when used solely for EC, the Cu-IUD becomes cost-effective after just 4 months of use, and can remain highly effective for more than 10 years.[2,22] Lack of counseling about Cu-IUD as an EC method, high upfront costs, insurance obstacles, and provider discomfort with same-day insertion are barriers to use.[90] Even among clinicians who routinely counseled patients on IUDs for general contraception, the Cu-IUD was unlikely to be discussed as an EC method.[29] New research indicates that women are interested in the use of Cu-IUD for EC. Of women presenting to clinics in Philadelphia and Utah to obtain EC or to take pregnancy tests, 12% to 15% of women would be interested in a Cu-IUD for EC if available.[1,26,79,91]

In addition to incorporating EC as a routine part of health care, increased attention must be placed on appropriate provision of EC after sexual assault.[92] Up to 5% of sexual assault survivors become pregnant from the assault.[93] In a population based-survey of US emergency departments, there was no increase in the provision of EC for sexual assault survivors between 2004 and 2009.[94] A 2013 study reported 40% of US hospitals did not provide EC to sexual assault survivors.[18,92] Objection to the provision of EC limits access, because of misinformation regarding its mechanism of action or broader objections to the provision of contraception.[79,87,92] Of hospitals that do provide EC, up to 30% prescribe the less-effective Yuzpe method.[8,79,95] All women who have experienced sexual assault should be offered effective EC in a timely manner to reduce the psychological and physical sequelae of rape-related pregnancy.

SUMMARY

EC provides women with a second chance to prevent pregnancy and should be regularly addressed during routine visits. Cu-IUD is the most effective method, followed by UPA, then LNG-ECP, and last the Yuzpe method. Advance provision alone is inadequate to optimize uptake of the ECP methods. Clinicians must strive to encourage state and federal agencies to enforce the current legislation, which provides women access to all FDA-approved contraceptive methods through the Affordable Care Act.

REFERENCES

1. Raymond E, Cleland K. Clinical practice. Emergency contraception. N Engl J Med 2015;372:14.
2. Trussell J, Leveque J, Koenig J, et al. The economic value of contraception: a comparison of 15 methods. Am J Public Health 1995;85:494–503.
3. Hatcher R, Trussell J, Nelson AL, et al, editors. Contraceptive technology. 20th revised edition. New York: Ardent Media; 2011.
4. Mosher WD, Jones J. Use of contraception in the United States: 1982-2008. Vital Health Stat 23 2010;(29):1–44.
5. Grimes D, Raymond E, Jones B. Emergency contraception over-the-counter: the medical and legal imperatives. Obstet Gynecol 2001;98(1):151–5.

6. Raymond EG, Weaver MA. Effect of an emergency contraceptive pill intervention on pregnancy risk behavior. Contraception 2008;77:333–6.

7. Weaver MA, Raymond EG, Baecher L. Attitude and behavior effects in a randomized trial of increased access to emergency contraception. Obstet Gynecol 2009; 103(1):107–16.

8. Raine TR, Harper CC, Rocca CH, et al. Direct access to emergency contraception through pharmacies and effect on unintended pregnancy and SITs: a randomized control trial. JAMA 2005;293:54–62.

9. Polis CB, Schaffer K, Blanchard K, et al. Advance provision of emergency contraception for pregnancy prevention (full review). Cochrane Database Syst Rev 2007;(2):CD005497.

10. Glasier A, Cameron S, Blithe D, et al. Can we identify women at risk of pregnancy despite using emergency contraception? Data from randomized trials of ulipristal acetate and levonorgestrel. Contraception 2011;84:363–7.

11. Wilcox A, Dunson D, Weinberg C, et al. Liklihood of conception with a single act of intercourse: providing benchmark rates for assessment of post-coital contraceptives. Contraception 2001;63:211–5.

12. Kapp N, Abitbol JL, Mathe H, et al. Effect of body weight and BMI on the efficacy of levonorgestrel contraception. Contraception 2015;91:97–104.

13. Raymond E, Taylor D, Trussell J, et al. Minimum effectiveness of the levonorgestrel regimen of emergency contraception. Contraception 2004;69: 79–81.

14. Cameron S, Glasier A. The need to take a "new look" at emergency contraception. J Fam Plann Reprod Health Care 2010;36(1):3–4.

15. Wilcox A, Weinberg C, Baird D. Timing of sexual intercourse in relation to ovulation. N Engl J Med 1995;333(23):1517–21.

16. Noe G, Croxatto HB, Salvatierra AM, et al. Contraceptive efficacy of emergency contraception with levonorgestrel given before or after ovulation. Contraception 2011;84(5):486–92.

17. Li D, Wilcox A, Dunson D. Benchmark pregnancy rates and the assessment of post-coital contraceptives: an update. Contraception 2015;91:344–9.

18. Westley E, Rich S, Lawton H. New research in emergency and postcoital contraception. Curr Obstet Gynecol Rep. Published online April 01, 2014. http://dx.doi.org/10.1007/s13669-014-0079-6. Accessed September 7, 2015.

19. Lundsberg L, Pal L, Gariepy A, et al. Knowledge, attitudes, and practices regarding conception and fertility: a population-based survey among reproductive-age United States women. Fertil Steril 2014;101(3):767–74.

20. Raymond EG, Stewart F, Weaver M, et al. Impact of increased access to emergency contraceptive pills: a randomized controlled trial. Obstet Gynecol 2006; 108:1098–106.

21. Trussell J, Guthrie K. Talking straight about emergency contraception. J Fam Plann Reprod Health Care 2007;33(3):139–42.

22. Trussell J, Raymond E, Cleland K. Emergency contraception: a last chance to prevent unintended pregnancy. Available at: http://ec.princeton.edu/questions/ec-review.pdf. Accessed May 8, 2015.

23. Wu S, Godfrey EM, Wojdyla D, et al. Copper T380A intrauterine device for emergency contraception: a prospective, multicenter, cohort clinical trial. BJOG 2010; 117:1205–10.

24. Cheng L, Che Y, Gulmezoglu AM. Interventions for emergency contraception. Cochrane Database Syst Rev 2012;(8):CD001324.

25. Cleland K, Zhu H, Goldstuck N, et al. The efficacy of intrauterine devices for emergency contraception: a systematic review of 35 years of experience. Humanit Rep 2012;27(7):1994–2000.

26. Turok DK, Godfrey EM, Wojdyla D, et al. Copper T380 intrauterine device for emergency contraception: highly effective at any time in the menstrual cycle. Humanit Rep 2013;28(10):2672–6.

27. Centers for Disease Control and Prevention. US Selected Practice Recommendations for Contraceptive Use, 2013: adapted from the World Health Organization Selected Practice Recommendations for Contraceptive Use, 2nd Edition. MMWR Recomm Rep 2013;62:1–60.

28. Zhou L, Xiao B. Emergency contraception with multiload CU-375 SL IUD: a multicenter clinical trial. Contraception 2001;64:107–12.

29. Harper C, Speidel J, Drey E, et al. Copper intrauterine device for contraception: clinical practice among contraceptive providers. Obstet Gynecol 2012;119:220–6.

30. Lalitkumar PGL, Berger C, Gemzell-Danielsson K. Emergency contraception. Best Pract Res Clin Endocrinol Metab 2013;27:91–101.

31. Gemzell-Danielsson K, Berger C, Lalitkumar PGL. Emergency contraception-mechanisms of action. Contraception 2013;87:300–8.

32. Stanford J, Mikolajczyk R. Mechanisms of action of intrauterine devices: update and estimation of postfertilization effects. Am J Obstet Gynecol 2002;187:1699–708.

33. Roblero L, Guadarrama A, Lopez T, et al. Effect of copper ion on the moltility, viability, acrosome reaction and fertilizing capacity of human spermatozoa in vitro. Reprod Fertil Dev 1996;8:871–4.

34. Ulmann G, Hammerstein J. Inhibition of sperm motility in vitro by copper wire. Contraception 1972;6:71–6.

35. Kesseru E, Camacho-Ortega P. Influence of metals on in vitro sperm migration in the human cervical mucus. Contraception 1972;6:231–40.

36. Hefnawi F, Kandil O, Askalani H, et al. Influence of the copper IUD and the Lippes loop on sperm migration in the human cervical mucus. Contraception 1975;11:541–7.

37. Hagenfeldt K, Johannisson E, Brenner P. Intrauterine contraception with the copper-T device. Effect upon endometrial, morphology. Contraception 1972;6:207–18.

38. Larsson B, Hamberger L. The concentration of copper in human uterine secretion during four years after insertion of a copper-containing intrauterine device. Fertil Steril 1977;28(6):624–6.

39. Wollen AL, Sandvei R, Skare A, et al. The localization and concentration of copper in the fallopian tube in women with or without an intrauterine contraceptive device. Acta Obstet Gynecol Scand 1994;73(3):195–9.

40. Larsson B, Lijung B, Hamberger L. The influence of copper on the in vitro motility of the human fallopian tube. Am J Obstet Gynecol 1976;125(5):682–90.

41. Ortiz M, Croxatto H. Copper-T intrauterine device and levonorgestrel intrauterine system: biological bases of their mechanism of action. Contraception 2007;75:S16–30.

42. National Collaborating Centre for Women's Health. Long-acting reversible contraception: the effective and appropriate use of long-acting reversible contraception. London: RCOG Press; 2005.

43. Centers for Disease Control and Prevention. US Medical Eligibility Criteria for Contraceptive Use, 2010. MMWR Recomm Rep 2010;59:50–1.

44. International Consortium for Emergency Contraception Policy Statement. The Intrauterine Device for Emergency Contraception. 2012. Available at: www.cecinof.org. Accessed March 27, 2015.

45. Mohllajee A, Curtis K, Peterson H. Does insertion and use of intrauterine device increase the risk of pelvic inflammatory disease among women with sexually transmitted infection? A systematic review. Contraception 2006;73:145–53.

46. Grimes D. Intrauterine device and upper-genital-tract infection. Lancet 2000;356: 1013–9.

47. Farley TM, Rosenberg MJ, Rowe PJ, et al. Intrauterine devices and pelvic inflammatory disease: an international perspective. Lancet 1992;339(8796):785–8.

48. Brahmi D, Steenland M, Renner RM, et al. Pregnancy outcomes with an IUD in situ: a systematic review. Contraception 2012;85:131–9.

49. World Health Organization. Mechanism of action, safety and efficacy of intrauterine devices. Report of a WHO Scientific Group. World Health Organ Tech Rep Ser 1987;753:1–91.

50. Blumenthal P, Voedisch A, Gemzell-Danielsson K. Strategies to prevent unintended pregnancy: increasing use of long-acting reversible contraception. Hum Reprod Update 2011;17(1):121–37.

51. Creinin M, Schlaff W, Archer D, et al. Progesterone receptor modulator for emergency contraception. Obstet Gynecol 2006;108:1089–97.

52. Glasier A, Cameron S, Fine P, et al. Ulipristal acetate versus levonorgestrel for emergency contraception: a randomized non-inferiority trial and meta analysis. Lancet 2010;375(9714):555–62.

53. Trussell J, Cleland K. Emergency contraceptive pill efficacy and BMI/body weight. Contraceptive technology. Available at: http://www.contraceptivetechnology.org/latebreakers/emergency-contraceptive-pill-efficacy-bmibody-weight/. Accessed July 22, 2015.

54. Brach V, Cochon L, Jesam C, et al. Immediate pre-ovulatory administration of 30 mg ulipristal acetate significantly delays follicular rupture. Hum Reprod 2010; 25(9):2256–63.

55. Croxatto HB, Brache V, Pavez M, et al. Pituitary-ovarian function following the standard levonorgestrel emergency contraceptive dose or a single 0.75-mg dose given on the days preceding ovulation. Contraception 2004;70:442–50.

56. Stratton P, Levens E, Hartog B, et al. Endometrial effects of a single early luteal dose of the selective progesterone receptor modulator CDB-2914. Fertil Steril 2010;93(6):2035–40.

57. Glasier A. Emergency contraception: clinical outcomes. Contraception 2013;87: 309–13.

58. Zinaman MJ, Clegg ED, Brown CC, et al. Estimates of human fertility and pregnancy loss. Fertil Steril 1996;65(3):503–9.

59. Ulipristal Acetate. [Package insert]. Available at: http://www.accessdata.fda.gov/drugsatfda_docs/label/2010/022474s000lbl.pdf. Accessed May 8, 2015.

60. Levy D, Jager M, Kapp N, et al. Ulipristal acetate for emergency contraception: postmarketing experience after use by more than 1 million women. Contraception 2014;89:431–3.

61. Orleans RJ. Clinical review. NDA22–474. Ella (ulipristal acetate 30 mg). US Food and Drug Administration; 2010. Available at: http://www.fda.gov/downloads/Drugs/DevelopmentApprovalProcess/DevelopmentResources/UCM295393.pdf. Accessed September 7, 2015.

62. Saav I, Fiala C, Hamalainen JM, et al. Medical abortion in lactating women: low levels of mifepristone in breast milk. Acta Obstet Gynecol Scand 2010;89(5):618–22.

63. Plan B Onestep. [Package insert]. Available at: http://www.accessdata.fda.gov/drugsatfda_docs/label/2009/021998lbl.pdf. Accessed May 8, 2015.
64. von Hertzen H, Piaggio G, Ding J, et al. Low dose mifepristone and two regimens of levonorgestrel for emergency contraception: a WHO multicenter randomized trial. Lancet 2002;360:1803–10.
65. Randomized controlled trial of levonorgestrel versus the Yuzpe regimen of combined oral contraceptives for emergency contraception. Task Force on Postovulatory Methods of Fertility Regulation. Lancet 1998;352:428–33.
66. Arowojolu AO, Okewole IA, Adekunle AO. Comparative evaluation of the effectiveness and safety of two regimens of levonorgestrel for emergency contraception in Nigerians. Contraception 2002;66:269–73.
67. Ngai SW, Fan S, Li S, et al. A randomized trial to compare 24h versus 12h double dose regimen of levonorgestrel for emergency contraception. Hum Reprod 2004; 20:307–11.
68. Ho PC, Kwan MS. A prospective randomized comparison of levonorgestrel with the Yuzpe regimen in post-coital contraception. Hum Reprod 1993;8: 389–92.
69. Wu S, Wang C, Wang Y, et al. A randomized, double blind, multicenter study on comparing levonorgestrel and mifepristone for emergency contraception. J Reprod Med 1999;8(Suppl 1):43–6.
70. Hamoda H, Ashok PW, Stalder C, et al. A randomized control trial of mifepristone (10 mg) and levonorgestrel for emergency contraception. Obstet Gynecol 2004; 104:1307–13.
71. Zhang L, Chen J, Wang Y, et al. Pregnancy outcome after levonorgestrel-only emergency contraception failure: a prospective cohort study. Hum Reprod 2009;24:1605–11.
72. Sambol NC, Harper CC, Kim L, et al. Pharmakokinetics of single dose levonorgestrel in adolescents. Contraception 2006;74:104–9.
73. Kook K, Gabelnick H, Duncan G. Pharmacokinetics of levonorgestrel 0.75 mg tablets. Contraception 2002;66:73–6.
74. Gainer E, Massai R, Lillo S, et al. Levonorgestrel pharmacokinetics in plasma and milk of lactating women who take 1.5 mg for emergency contraception. Hum Reprod 2007;22(6):1578–84.
75. Batur P. Emergency contraception: separating fact from fiction. Cleve Clin J Med 2012;79(11):771–6.
76. International Consortium for Emergency Contraception. Using oral birth control pills as EC. 2014. Available at: www.cecinof.org. Accessed March 27, 2015.
77. von Hertzen H, Piaggio G. Emergency contraception with levonorgestrel or the Yuzpe regimen. Lancet 1939;1998:352.
78. Raman-Wilms L, Tseng AL, Wighardt S, et al. Fetal genital effects of first-trimester sex hormone exposure: a meta-analysis. Obstet Gynecol 1995; 85(1):141–9.
79. American College of Obsetricians and Gynecologists. ACOG committee opinion no. 542: access to emergency contraception. Obstet Gynecol 2012; 120:1250–3.
80. Committee on Adolescence. Emergency contraception. Pediatrics 2005;116: 1026.
81. Stream G. American Academy of Family Physicians Statement: AAFP Opposes U.S. Department of Justice's Appeal of Emergency Contraception Ruling. [Press Release]. Available at: http://www.aafp.org/media-center/releases-statements/all/2013/contraception-planb.html. Accessed May 13, 2015.

82. American Academy of Pediatrics, American College of Obstetricians and Gyne-
    cologists, and Society of Adolescent Health and Medicine. Medical groups
    denounce HHS decision on access to emergency contraception: move defies
    strong evidence that emergency contraception is a safe, effective tool to prevent
    unintended pregnancy. [Press Release]. 2011. Available at: http://www.acog.org/
    ~/media/News%20Releases/20111207Release.ashx. Accessed May 13, 2015.
83. Association of Reproductive Health Professionals. Available at: https://www.arhp.
    org/about-us/position-statements. Accessed May 13, 2015.
84. American Public Health Association. Support of public education about emer-
    gency contraception and reduction or elimination of barriers to access. Policy
    Date: 11/18/2003 Policy Number: 200315. Available at: http://www.apha.org/
    policies-and-advocacy/public-health-policy-statements/policy-database/2014/
    07/24/15/29/support-of-public-ed-about-emergency-contraception-and-elimination-
    of-barriers-to-access. Accessed May 13, 2015.
85. Mackin ML, Clark K. Emergency contraception in Iowa pharmacies before and
    after over-the-counter approval. Public Health Nurs 2011;28:317–24.
86. Bayer LL, Edelman A, Caughey AB, et al. The price of emergency contraception
    in the United States: what is the cost-effectiveness of ulipristal acetate versus
    single-dose levonorgestrel? Contraception 2013;87(3):385–90.
87. Association of Reproductive Health Professionals (ARHP). 2011 Update on emer-
    gency contraception. Curricula Organizer for Reproductive Health Education
    (CORE). Available at: http://www.arhp.org/uploadDocs/CPECUpdate.pdf. Ac-
    cessed May 13, 2015.
88. Brant A, White K, St. Marie P. Pharmacy availability of ulipristal acetate emer-
    gency contraception: an audit study. Contraception 2014;90(3):338–9.
89. Wilkinson TA, Vargas G, Fahey N, et al. "I'll see what I can do": What adolescents
    experience when requesting emergency contraception. J Adolesc Health 2014;
    54(1):14–9.
90. Thompson K, Belden P. Counseling for emergency contraception: time for a
    tiered approach. Available at: www.arhp.org. Accessed April 12, 2015.
91. Schwarz E, Kavanaugh M, Douglas E, et al. Interest in intrauterine contraception
    among seekers of emergency contraception and pregnancy testing. Obstet Gy-
    necol 2009;113(4):833–9.
92. Patel A, Roston A, Tilmon S, et al. Assessing the extent of provision of compre-
    hensive medical care management for female sexual assault patients in US hos-
    pital emergency departments. Int J Gynaecol Obstet 2013;123(1):24–8.
93. Holmes MM, Resnick HS, Kilpatrick GG, et al. Rape-related pregnancy: estimates
    and descriptive characteristics from a national sample of women. Am J Obstet
    Gynecol 1996;175(2):320–5.
94. Patel A, Tilmon S, Bhogireddy V, et al. Emergency contraception after sexual as-
    sault: changes in provision from 2004-2009. J Reprod Med 2012;57(3–4):98–104.
95. Bakhru A, Mallinger JB, Fox MC. Postexposure prophylaxis for victims of sexual
    assault: treatments and attitudes of emergency department physicians. Contra-
    ception 2010;82(2):168–73.

Sterilization
A Review and Update

 CrossMark

Chailee Moss, MD[a], Michelle M. Isley, MD, MPH[b],*

KEYWORDS

- Sterilization • Tubal • Female • Male • Laparoscopy • Hysteroscopy
- Postpartum • Interval

KEY POINTS

- Sterilization is one of the most frequently used methods of contraception in the United States and worldwide, with a female-to-male sterilization ratio of 3 to 1.
- Female sterilization can be performed using an abdominal approach or via laparoscopy or hysteroscopy.
- The cumulative 10-year failure rate for all methods is 18.5 per 1000 procedures; postpartum partial salpingectomy has the lowest 10-year failure rate and bipolar coagulation the highest.
- Sterilization should be considered a permanent form of contraception. Long-acting reversible methods of contraception, such as the intrauterine device and the implant, are as effective as permanent sterilization, but reversible.
- Vasectomy is a safe and highly effective method of sterilization.

INTRODUCTION

Sterilization is one of the most frequently used methods of contraception worldwide. The recent National Survey of Family Growth reveals that among women aged 15 to 44 years in the United States, 15.5% rely on female and 5.1% rely on male sterilization.[1] Use of sterilization varies by age and race/ethnicity. Among women aged 35 to 44 years, nearly one in three rely on female sterilization, compared with less than 1% of women age 15 to 24 years. Of non-Hispanic black women, 21.3% rely on female sterilization, compared with 18.8% of Hispanic women, and 14.0% of non-Hispanic white women. The latest National Survey of Family Growth also found that the use of female sterilization declines with greater educational attainment.

Author Disclosure: Dr C. Moss has no disclosures. Dr M.M. Isley is a trainer for Nexplanon (Merck). She is also in the speaker bureau for Liletta (Actavis Pharma).
[a] Department of Obstetrics and Gynecology, Ohio State University, 395 West 12th Avenue, Columbus, OH 43210, USA; [b] Department of Obstetrics and Gynecology, Ohio State University, 395 West 12th Avenue, Room 503, Columbus, OH 43210, USA
* Corresponding author.
E-mail address: Michelle.Isley@osumc.edu

Obstet Gynecol Clin N Am 42 (2015) 713–724
http://dx.doi.org/10.1016/j.ogc.2015.07.003
0889-8545/15/$ – see front matter © 2015 Elsevier Inc. All rights reserved.

Since 1995, a decline in rates of female sterilization has been noted.[2] This is hypothesized to be a result of demographic, economic, social, and cultural factors, such as delayed childbirth and improved access to and use of long-acting reversible contraceptive methods.[2] Despite the decline, female tubal sterilization is one of the most commonly performed gynecologic surgeries, after cesarean section and abortion.[3]

Female sterilization can be performed using an abdominal approach or via laparoscopy or hysteroscopy. Sterilization approach will vary based on timing. It can be performed immediately postpartum, or as an interval procedure, unrelated to a pregnancy. Approximately 50% of female sterilizations are performed immediately postpartum. Sterilization follows 8% to 9% of live births, most often at the time of cesarean delivery.[2] Since 1995 and the adoption of laparoscopy, interval sterilizations have become more common and have shifted the procedure from the inpatient to the ambulatory setting.[4] Because of the ease of sterilization in the ambulatory setting, there has been a dramatic increase in the number of interval procedures performed in the United States, from a rate of 0.4 sterilizations per 1000 unsterilized women in 1980 to a rate of 6.4 sterilizations per 1000 unsterilized women at its peak in 1996.[2] The choice and time of sterilization are affected by individual patient preference, medical assessment of acute risk, access to services, and insurance coverage. Current methods of female sterilization include mechanical occlusion of the fallopian tubes, coagulation, and tubal excision.

Much of what is known about sterilization risks, failure rates, and regret comes from the US Collaborative Review of Sterilization (CREST) Study. This was a large prospective cohort study in US academic medical centers that enrolled over 12,000 women who underwent sterilization and then followed the women for more than 10 years. In the CREST study, the cumulative 10-year failure rate for all methods was 18.5 failures per 1000 procedures.[5] Failure rates for each specific sterilization method can be found in **Table 1**.

FEMALE STERILIZATION: LAPAROSCOPY

Laparoscopic sterilization has a number of advantages and disadvantages (**Table 2**). It is typically performed as an ambulatory surgery, with women going home a few hours

Table 1
Sterilization failure rate by type of procedure performed; ectopic pregnancy risk

Method	Failures, Year 1 Per 1000 Procedures	Failures, Year 10 Per 1000 Procedures	Ectopic Pregnancies, Year 10 Per 1000 Procedures
Bipolar	2.3	24.8	17.1
Monopolar	0.7	7.5	1.8
Silastic rings	5.9	17.7	7.3
Hulka clips	18.2	36.5	8.5
Postpartum partial salpingectomy	0.6	7.5	1.5
All methods	5.5	18.5	7.3

Data from Peterson HB, Xia Z, Hughes JM, et al. The risk of pregnancy after tubal sterilization: findings from the U.S. Collaborative Review of Sterilization. Am J Obstet Gynecol 1996;174:1161–8; and Peterson HB, Xia Z, Hughes JM, et al. The risk for ectopic pregnancy after tubal sterilization. N Engl J Med 1997;336:762–7.

Table 2
Advantages and disadvantages of different approaches to sterilization

Abdominal	Laparoscopic	Via Hysteroscopy
Opportunity to inspect abdominal and pelvic organs	Opportunity to inspect abdominal and pelvic organs	Opportunity to inspect uterine cavity
Small incision	Small incision	No incision
Immediately effective	Immediately effective	Effective after 3 mo
Local, general, or spinal anesthesia	General anesthesia	Local or general anesthesia
Operating room setting	Operating room setting	Office or operating room setting

after surgery is completed. The overall complication rate for laparoscopic sterilization is 0.4% to 1%. Not all women are good candidates for laparoscopic surgery, with surgical complication risk independently related to diabetes, previous abdominal or pelvic surgery, and obesity. Traditionally, methods of laparoscopic sterilization have been electrocoagulation and mechanical tubal occlusion. Because of the new interest in the role the fallopian tube may play in the development of ovarian cancer, laparoscopic sterilization may also be accomplished by performing bilateral salpingectomy (see section on opportunistic salpingectomy). Laparoscopic sterilization is normally performed as an interval procedure, but it can also be performed after a spontaneous or induced abortion without risk of increased complication.[6]

Electrocoagulation

The earliest laparoscopic sterilization methods employed electrocoagulation. With electrocoagulation, a 3 cm section of the isthmic portion of the fallopian tube is completely coagulated. Electrocoagulation can be accomplished with unipolar or bipolar energy, both of which carry the risk of thermal injury to adjacent structures.

In the CREST study, unipolar coagulation had the lowest failure rate for interval methods but is no longer used because of the risk of conductive thermal injury. Bipolar coagulation is used almost exclusively for sterilization with electrocoagulation, because the risk of thermal injury is lower with this technology. In a retrospective study comparing 846 silastic ring sterilizations with 4500 electrocautery sterilizations, 13 cases of electrical burns were reported for electrocautery cases, resulting in 3 bowel resections. No additional surgeries were required in the silastic ring group. The rate of pelvic infection was also higher in the electrocautery group (15 cases), whereas no infections were identified in the ring procedure group.[7]

The 10-year cumulative failure rate for monopolar electrocoagulation is 7.5 failures per 1000 procedures.[5] The 10-year cumulative failure rate for bipolar electrocoagulation is 24.8 failures per 1000 procedures.[5] Sterilization failures occur with bipolar electrocoagulation when there is incomplete desiccation of the fallopian tube endosalpinx.[8] Methods to decrease the high rates of failure with bipolar sterilization include use of more than 25 W of current in cutting mode, use of an inline current meter to ensure the appropriate energy is delivered, and coagulation of 3 or more sites of the fallopian tube.[9,10]

Mechanical Occlusion

Mechanical techniques for laparoscopic sterilization use devices such as clips or rings to permanently obstruct the lumen of the fallopian tube. The Falope-ring (Gyrus, Southborough, Massachusetts) is a silicone plastic (silastic) band. Using a special applicator, a 2 cm to 3 cm segment of the tube is drawn up into the applicator, and the silastic band is released onto the tubal loop. The silastic band constricts the loop and blocks the tube. Over time, the constricted loop, deprived of its blood supply, will undergo necrosis, healing, fibrosis, and finally occlusion. The 10-year cumulative failure rate for the silastic band is 17.7 failures per 1000 procedures.[5]

Filshie (CooperSurgical, Trumbull, Connecticut) clips are silicone-lined titanium clips that are placed around the fallopian tubes to cause occlusion. The clip is placed approximately 3 cm from the cornua, and both sides of the tube are visualized to ensure the entire tube is crushed and occluded by the clip. Filshie clips were not included in the CREST study. The Filshie clip was subsequently approved for use based on prospective trials demonstrating efficacy equal to that of other methods at 2 years (9.7 failures per 1000 procedures).[11]

A second type of occlusive clip, the Hulka (Richard Wolf Medical Instruments Corporation, Vernon Hills, Illinois) clip, is a hinged spring clip that is placed over the isthmic portion of the tube. The spring-loaded clip is unpopular and rarely used because of its high failure rates (36.5 failures per 1000 procedures).[5]

Comparison of Laparoscopic Sterilization Techniques

Several studies have compared laparoscopic sterilization methods, and conclusions differ. Bhiwandiwala and colleagues[12] compared electrocoagulation, the silastic ring, and the spring-loaded clip and found that there was no difference in surgical difficulty, surgical complications, or rates of technical failures. In another study comparing methods, although total complication rates were similar with all methods, bleeding from the tubes and wound and pelvic infections were more frequent with the silastic ring.[13] In the most recent comparison by Khandwala,[14] technical difficulties and technical failures occurred less often with bipolar coagulation than with the ring or clip (Hulka and Filshie), but more serious complications occurred with bipolar coagulation (electrical burns). The greater technical difficulties and failures with clips and rings were caused by problems in applying the devices in the setting of tuboperitoneal pathology. Compared with the ring, both types of clips were associated with fewer complications. In women who underwent subsequent tubal reversal, pregnancy rates were highest after sterilization with clips. The authors concluded that bipolar coagulation is preferable in women with pelvic adhesions and tubal pathology and that clips are preferred in women who may be candidates for future sterilization reversal.[14]

Laparoscopic Sterilization Adverse Effects

Care has been taken to investigate anecdotal reports of a constellation of complaints after tubal sterilization, including menstrual irregularities, pelvic pain, and worsened premenstrual symptoms, sometimes called post-tubal sterilization syndrome. One review identified over 200 articles on the topic and concluded from the most relevant that tubal sterilization is not associated with an increased risk of menstrual dysfunction, dysmenorrhea, or increased premenstrual distress in women who undergo the procedure after the age of 30 years. Women younger than 30 years with a history of menstrual dysfunction before the tubal sterilization may be at a slightly increased risk.[15] The follow-up data from the CREST study revealed that women who had undergone tubal sterilization were no more likely than other women to have menstrual abnormalities.[16]

Tubal Sterilization Failure After Laparoscopic Sterilization

Tubal ligation failure is a significant concern for patients, not only because of the social and economic consequences of unintended pregnancy, but also because of the increased risk of ectopic pregnancy. Soderstrom[8] performed surgical and pathologic examination on 47 cases of repeat sterilization to determine cause of failure. In cases of mechanical occlusion devices, sterilization failure was caused by defective devices, improper device placement technique, or devices that were placed in an improper location. Bipolar coagulation sterilization failure resulted from incomplete tissue damage and viable endosalpinx.[8] A study of tubal ligation failures in procedures performed by residents showed that most postocclusion pregnancies occurred because of improper application of sterilization silastic rings or clips, with clips being placed on the round ligament and/or devices being deployed improperly so as to incompletely occlude the tubal lumen.[17] Thus, care should be taken to identify tubal fimbriae to avoid application to the round ligaments, and to completely deploy occlusive devices.

FEMALE STERILIZATION: OPEN ABDOMINAL METHODS

The postpartum period is a convenient time for tubal ligation in women who desire sterilization, because it can be performed in conjunction with cesarean delivery or within the first 24 to 48 hours after delivery. Sterilization in the immediate period after a vaginal delivery takes advantage of the enlarged postpartum uterus; the size of a recently gravid uterus improves fallopian tube proximity to the umbilicus. Thus, a small infra- or supraumbilical minilaparotomy incision can be made to easily access the tube with minimal trauma and cosmetic deficit from the resulting scar and rarely prolongs hospitalization. Cesarean section is an ideal setting for sterilization because of the wide operative field and ease of access to the fallopian tubes. Rarely, significant adhesive disease prevents identification of and access to the tubes.

At the time of a postpartum sterilization, a tubal excision procedure, most often a partial salpingectomy, is performed. Methods of partial salpingectomy include the Pomeroy, Parkland, Uchida, and Irving. Application of Filshie clips for postpartum sterilization is reported; however, several studies have demonstrated that, compared with partial salpingectomy, the clips are significantly less effective.[18,19] Postpartum partial salpingectomy is the most effective method of sterilization, with a 10-year cumulative failure rate of 7.5 failures per 1000 procedures.[5]

In developing countries, interval minilaparotomy with partial salpingectomy may be the most common approach because of limited resources for purchase and upkeep of laparoscopic equipment. Interval minilaparotomy can be performed on an outpatient basis using local anesthesia. Compared with laparoscopy, minilaparotomy carries no increased risk for major morbidity and a slightly increased risk for minor morbidity.[20]

OPPORTUNISTIC SALPINGECTOMY

The findings of premalignant cells in the epithelium of the fallopian tube has led to theories of a tubal origin of ovarian cancer and the hypothesis that salpingectomy may decrease ovarian cancer risk.[21] Bilateral complete salpingectomy is now being considered as a method of sterilization that could potentially decrease ovarian cancer risk.

Salpingectomy can be performed as an open procedure or via laparoscopy. Theoretically, bilateral salpingectomy is 100% effective, although at least 1 case report describes a pregnancy after bilateral tubal removal.[22] Salpingectomy is the preferred method for women who have become pregnant after a tubal ligation.[23]

Several case–control studies published in the 1980s demonstrated a protective effect of tubal occlusion against ovarian cancer.[24] A recent pooled analysis of 13 case–control studies demonstrated a 29% decreased risk of invasive ovarian cancers in women who had undergone tubal sterilization.[25] To date, there have been no long-term prospective data demonstrating that bilateral salpingectomy results in a larger reduction of ovarian cancer risk compared with tubal occlusion alone.

Concerns about routine opportunistic salpingectomy include higher surgical morbidity and a higher risk for premature menopause through impaired vascular supply to the ovaries.[26] Data regarding ovarian function after salpingectomy performed during hysterectomy appear reassuring.[25,27,28] Much of the data about surgical risk associated with salpingectomy comes from studies examining surgical outcomes and complications of prophylactic salpingectomy at the time of benign hysterectomy. These studies reveal no difference in average operating time, estimated blood loss, intraoperative complications, and postoperative complications.[29,30] One study specifically compared tubal ligation with bilateral salpingectomy, including open postpartum salpingectomy and salpingectomy done at the time of cesarean section.[31] Investigators found that compared with tubal ligation, bilateral salpingectomy increased operating room time by 10.2 minutes but did not increase length of hospital stay. There was also no increased risk for hospital readmission or blood transfusion in the bilateral salpingectomy group.[31]

Thus, in women undergoing tubal ligation for purposes of sterilization, counseling should include a discussion of complete fallopian tube removal, or opportunistic salpingectomy. The procedure may be especially appealing to women with an increased risk of ovarian cancer. Women should be informed that the potential benefit is theoretic and that there is the potential for increased surgical risks and compromised ovarian blood supply leading to premature menopause. Additionally, women considering complete salpingectomy need to be informed that they will not have the option of tubal reversal, and that although data appear reassuring on ovarian function after the procedure, the evidence is limited.[32]

FEMALE STERILIZATION: TRANSCERVICAL

Transcervical sterilization offers the practitioner the advantage of avoiding abdominal incisions, limiting infection risk, and minimizing equipment requirements and anesthesia. Methods have included thermal occlusion, silicon plugs formed in situ, and instilling sclerosing agents into the uterus. In the case of thermal agents, risk to bowel and bladder injury was significant; in the case of other blindly instilled agents, risks of extravasation and migration were notable flaws. The shortcomings of early approaches ultimately limited its appeal as safe and effective laparoscopic techniques developed. The advancement of hysteroscopy has allowed practitioners to directly visualize fallopian tube ostia and approach transcervical sterilization in a targeted manner.

Placement of Microinserts via Hysteroscopy

Essure (Bayer HealthCare Pharmaceuticals Incorporated, Whippany, New Jersey) is a US Food and Drug Administration (FDA) approved method of sterilization via hysteroscopy available in the United States. Essure microinserts are placed into each fallopian tube using a proprietary deployment device under direct visualization. Advantages of this procedure include no incisions and no entry into the abdominal cavity, option to perform in the outpatient setting, and avoidance of general anesthesia. The Essure microinserts are made of titanium, stainless steel, nickel, and Dacron fibers that induce an inflammatory response and fibrotic occlusion of the intramural lumen of the fallopian tube.[33] A disadvantage of this type of sterilization is that it is not immediately effective. Because tubal fibrosis occurs over time, interim contraception should be used until a 3-month postprocedure hysterosalpingogram (HSG) can be performed to confirm bilateral tubal occlusion.

Placement of bilateral microinserts into the tubes during hysteroscopy is not always possible. Using published studies, Gariepy and colleagues[34] estimated the probability of successful sterilization via laparoscopy or hysteroscopy. The proportion of women having a successful sterilization procedure on the first attempt is 88% for Essure done via hysteroscopy in the operating room and 87% for an office-based Essure procedure, compared with 99% for laparoscopic sterilization. At 1 year, the probability of having any successful sterilization procedure within 1 year was 99% for women starting with laparoscopic sterilization, 95% for women starting with an Essure procedure in the operating room, and 94% for women starting with a procedure in the office. In this study, not all women who selected Essure were ultimately sterilized by this method. Approximately 12% of the women who initially attempted sterilization via hysteroscopy ultimately achieved sterilization via laparoscopy.[34] Published Essure placement success rates often do not include women who failed an initial attempt at microinsert placement or women who failed to return for the HSG, which falsely elevates the percentage of successful sterilizations.

Patient counseling that includes accurate successful sterilization rates is imperative. For women selecting Essure, 85% to 86% will have a successful sterilization procedure by 3 months.[34] Poor visualization of the tubal ostia or a history of any sexually transmitted infection may increase the risk for microinsert placement failure.[35,36] Successful placement is not significantly related to parity, premedication with nonsteroidal anti-inflammatory medications, mode of analgesia, or combination with another procedure.[35]

Once tubal occlusion is confirmed with HSG, the chance of pregnancy following Essure is low.[37] One 5-year follow-up study reported a failure rate of 0.25%.[38] Clinical experience with Essure has demonstrated significantly more loss to follow-up for the confirmatory HSG than expected. Compliance with the required follow-up HSG varies, from 13% to 94%.[39–41] Barriers to adherence to the HSG include scheduling, insurance coverage, and equipment limitations.

There is a small risk of an allergic reaction to the inserts in patients with nickel hypersensitivity, although in clinical practice this is incredibly rare (0.01%). Symptoms reported with nickel hypersensitivity appear to be mild and do not necessarily resolve with implant removal.[42] At the present time, patients who have an allergy to HSG contrast dye should be counseled on alternate methods of contraception, as HSG is currently the gold standard method of confirming tubal occlusion after placement. Several investigators have suggested the possibility of more comfortable, less expensive modalities to confirm Essure placement, including ultrasound and radiograph, but none is approved at this time in the United States.

STERILIZATION COUNSELING

All counseling about sterilization should begin with a discussion of the full range of contraceptive options, which include methods of female sterilization, vasectomy, as well as long-acting reversible contraceptive methods (intrauterine devices and implants), since these methods are as effective as sterilization but reversible. In preparation for any permanent sterilization, a patient should be counseled on the intentionally irreversible nature of the procedure. In the CREST study, the cumulative risk of regret over 14 years of follow-up was 12.7%. Age was a risk factor for regret; risk of regret for women aged 30 or younger was 20.3%, while the risk for women over the age of 30 was 5.9%.[43] Other risk factors for regret after sterilization are having less information about the procedure, having less access to information about or support for use of an alternative contraceptive method, and having made the decision due to partner pressure or because of a medical indication.[44] Time and care should be taken when counseling about sterilization. Women who are unsure about future childbearing should be strongly counseled to consider a long-acting reversible type of contraception.

As with any nonbarrier contraceptive method, sterilization does not protect against sexually transmitted infections (STIs), and all patients should be counseled on condom use for STI protection.

STERILIZATION FAILURE

Although sterilization is an excellent method of contraception, all methods of sterilization have a risk of failure (see **Table 1**). Failure rates are age dependent; the younger the woman is at time of sterilization, the more likely she is to have a sterilization failure.[5] When sterilization fails, there is an increased risk of ectopic pregnancy. Risk of ectopic pregnancy also varies by sterilization method (see **Table 1**). Using the CREST data, at 10 years after sterilization, the overall risk of ectopic pregnancy for all methods was 7.3 cases per 1000 procedures.[45] The highest risk for ectopic pregnancy was for bipolar coagulation, with 17.1 ectopic pregnancies identified per 1000 procedures at 10 years. Women younger than 30 years old who undergo bipolar coagulation sterilization were 27 times more likely to have an ectopic pregnancy than those who had a postpartum salpingectomy.[10] Thus, patients should be counseled to seek immediate medical attention after their sterilization if they experience a positive pregnancy test, symptoms of pregnancy, or significant abdominal pain.

STERILIZATION CONTRAINDICATIONS

Medical comorbidities must be considered prior to undertaking any sterilization procedure. Although sterilization via laparoscopy and hysteroscopy are relatively short procedures, patients with significant contraindication to anesthesia or positioning during procedures should be counseled on alternate methods of contraception or sterilization of male partners.

Obesity is sometimes cited as a contraindication to immediate postpartum tubal sterilization by minilaparotomy, because adipose tissue can limit access to the uterine fundus and the fallopian tubes. However, problems of central obesity can be alleviated by extension of the infra- or supraumbilical incision at the time of surgery. Morbid obesity can also limit laparoscopic approaches by preventing adequate ventilation or positioning in Trendelenburg. Hysteroscopy may be the preferred approach in these patients.

Adhesive disease from prior abdominal surgeries can pose a significant challenge during tubal occlusion, both with laparoscopy and with open surgeries at the time of cesarean or immediately postpartum. Patients with extensive history of abdominal surgery should be counseled on the possibility that their fallopian tubes may not be accessible at the time of abdominal or laparoscopic surgery, and they might require alternative methods of birth control. In these cases, sterilization via hysteroscopy or long-acting reversible contraceptive devices may be recommended.

MALE STERILIZATION

Vasectomy is the least invasive technique for sterilization and should always be included in the discussion about permanent birth control methods. With vasectomy, the vas deferens is ligated via a small scrotal incision in an outpatient setting with local anesthesia. Particular consideration of this method should be undertaken in counseling women for whom operative or procedural risks of sterilization or pregnancy are prohibitive. Vasectomy has the advantage of avoiding potential pelvic organ injury or risk for ectopic pregnancy.

Vasectomy is a highly effective method, with a failure rate of 0.10% to 0.15%.[46] Vasectomy does not have adverse consequences to health or cause sexual side effects.[47] Complications are rare and include bleeding and hematoma formation, infection, and granuloma formation. Because residual sperm remain in the vas deferens beyond the point of occlusion, vasectomy is not immediately effective, and another form of contraception should be used until azospermia can be confirmed. At 3 months and 11 to 20 ejaculations, 80% of men will have azospermia.[48]

STERILIZATION REVERSAL

Although sterilization is meant to be permanent, some women will express regret and request sterilization reversal. Approximately 1% to 3% of women will seek reversal at a later date.[49] Factors related to seeking tubal reversal include sterilization at a young age, sterilization done at the time of cesarean delivery or immediately postpartum, or a change in relationship status.[50] These patients may pursue surgery to reconnect ligated fallopian tubes. Pregnancy rates after tubal ligation reversal range from 31% to 88%.[51] Several factors affect the pregnancy rate after sterilization reversal.[52] Age is a significant factor, with a higher pregnancy rate for women younger than 36 years. Higher pregnancy rates are seen after clips (78%) or silastic rings (72%), compared with coagulation (68%) or the Pomeroy partial salpingectomy method (67%), but differences in pregnancy rates were not significant.[52] Tubal length is controversial, but some studies have demonstrated a tubal length greater than 4 cm improves pregnancy rates.[50,53] In vitro fertilization is also an option for patients desiring fertility after tubal sterilization. These patients can be referred to a reproductive endocrinologist for further evaluation and counseling. After vasectomy reversal via vasovasostomy, pregnancy rates range from 33% to 64%.[54–56]

STERILIZATION COST

Vasectomy is one of the most cost-effective methods of contraception.[57] At an estimated $710 per procedure, vasectomy is one-fourth the cost of tubal ligation ($2912).[57] If female sterilization is done as an office-based procedure, expected costs are less, with estimates of $2367.[58]

SUMMARY

Sterilization is a popular and highly effective method of contraception. Female sterilization can be performed as an abdominal procedure or via laparoscopy or hysteroscopy. Each approach has benefits and disadvantages, and patient characteristics and desires will determine the type and timing of the sterilization procedure performed. Counseling for sterilization should emphasize its permanence, and include discussion of both male and female sterilization as well as the highly effective but reversible long-acting contraceptive methods (IUDs, implant).

REFERENCES

1. Daniels K, Daugherty J, Jones J. Current contraceptive status among women aged 15-44: United States, 2011-2013. NCHS Data Brief 2014;173:1–8.

2. Chan LM, Westhoff CL. Tubal sterilization trends in the United States. Fertil Steril 2010;94:1–6.
3. Cullen KA, Hall MJ, Golosinsky A. Ambulatory surgery in the United States, 2006. Natl Health Stat Report 2009;11:1–25.
4. Pollack AE, Konnin LM, Haws JM, et al. Postpartum tubal sterilization in the United States, 1988–1994 [abstract]. 1997: Presented at the 1997 APHA Annual Meeting. Indianapolis, IN, November 9-13, 1997.
5. Peterson HB, Xia Z, Hughes JM, et al. The risk of pregnancy after tubal sterilization: findings from the U.S. Collaborative Review of Sterilization. Am J Obstet Gynecol 1996;174:1161–8.
6. Akhter HH, Flock ML, Rubin GL. Safety of abortion and tubal sterilization performed separately versus concurrently. Am J Obstet Gynecol 1985;152:619–23.
7. Baggish MS, Lee WK, Miro SJ, et al. Complications of laparoscopic sterilization. Comparison of 2 methods. Obstet Gynecol 1979;54:54–9.
8. Soderstrom RM. Sterilization failures and their causes. Am J Obstet Gynecol 1985;152:395–403.
9. Soderstrom RM, Levy BS, Engel T. Reducing bipolar sterilization failures. Obstet Gynecol 1989;74:60–3.
10. Peterson HB, Xia Z, Wilcox LS, et al. Pregnancy after tubal sterilization with bipolar electrocoagulation. U.S. Collaborative Review of Sterilization Working Group. Obstet Gynecol 1999;94:163–7.
11. Dominik R, Gates D, Sokal D, et al. Two randomized controlled trials comparing the Hulka and Filshie clips for sterilization. Contraception 2000;62:169–75.
12. Bhiwandiwala PP, Memford SD, Feldblum PJ. A comparison of different laparoscopic sterilization occlusion techniques in 24439 procedures. Am J Obstet Gynecol 1982;144:309–31.
13. Brenner WE. Evaluation of contemporary female sterilization methods. J Reprod Med 1981;26:439–53.
14. Khandwala SD. Laparoscopic sterilization: a comparison of current techniques. J Reprod Med 1988;33:463–6.
15. Gentile GP, Kaufman SC, Helbig DW. Is there any evidence for a post-tubal sterilization syndrome? Fertil Steril 1998;69:179–86.
16. Peterson HB, Jeng G, Folger SG, et al. The risk of menstrual abnormalities after tubal sterilization. U.S. Collaborative Review of Sterilization Working Group. N Engl J Med 2000;343:1681–7.
17. Stovall TG, Ling FW, O'Kelly KR, et al. Gross and histologic examination of tubal ligation failures in a residency training program. Obstet Gynecol 1990;76:461–5.
18. Rodriguez MI, Edelman AB, Kapp N. Postpartum sterilization with the titanium clip: a systematic review. Obstet Gynecol 2011;118:143–7 [Erratum appears in Obstet Gynecol 2011;188:961].
19. Rodriguez M, Seuc A, Sokal D. Comparative efficacy of postpartum sterilization with the titanium clip versus partial salpingectomy: a randomized controlled trial. BJOG 2013;120(1):108–12.
20. Kulier R, Boulvain M, Walker D, et al. Minilaparotomy and endoscopic techniques for tubal sterilization. Cochrane Database Syst Rev 2004;(3):CD001328.
21. Erickson BK, Conner MG, Landen CN Jr. The role of the fallopian tube in the origin on ovarian cancer. Am J Obstet Gynecol 2013;209:409–14.
22. Bollapragada SS, Bandyopadhyay S, Serle E, et al. Spontaneous pregnancy after bilateral salpingectomy. Fertil Steril 2005;83:767–8.
23. Chakravarti S, Shardlow J. Tubal pregnancy after sterilization. Br J Obstet Gynaecol 1975;82:58–60.

24. Cibula D, Widschwendter M, Majek O, et al. Tubal ligation and the risk of ovarian cancer: review and meta-analysis. Hum Reprod Update 2011;17:55–67.
25. Sieh W, Salvador S, McGuire V, et al. Tubal ligation and risk of ovarian cancer subtypes: a pooled analysis of case-control studies. Int J Epidemiol 2013;42: 579–89.
26. Polcher M, Hauptmann S, Fotopoulou C, et al. Opportunistic salpingectomies for the prevention of a high-grade serous carcinoma: a statement by the Kommission Ovar of the AGO. Arch Gynecol Obstet 2015;292:231–4.
27. Sezik M, Ozkaya O, Demir F, et al. Total salpingectomy during abdominal hysterectomy: effects on ovarian reserve and ovarian stromal blood flow. J Obstet Gynaecol Res 2007;33:863–9.
28. Findley AD, Siedhoff MT, Hobbs KA, et al. Short-term effects of salpingectomy during laparoscopic hysterectomy on ovarian reserve: a pilot randomized controlled trial. Fertil Steril 2013;100:1704–8.
29. Minig L, Chuang L, Patrono MG, et al. Surgical outcomes and complications of prophylactic salpingectomy at the time of benign hysterectomy in premenopausal women. J Minim Invasive Gynecol 2015;22:253–7.
30. Vorwergk J, Radosa MP, Nicolaus K, et al. Prophylactic bilateral salpingectomy (PBS) to reduce ovarian cancer risk incorporated in standard premenopausal hysterectomy: complications and re-operation rate. J Cancer Res Clin Oncol 2014;140:859–65.
31. McAlpine JN, Hanley GE, Woo MM, et al. Opportunistic salpingectomy: uptake, risks, and complications of a regional initiative for ovarian cancer prevention. Am J Obstet Gynecol 2014;210:471.e1–11.
32. Morelli M, Venturella R, Mocciaro R, et al. Prophylactic salpingectomy in premenopausal low-risk women for ovarian cancer: primum no nocere. Gyncol Oncol 2013;129:448–51.
33. Ubeda A, Labastida R, Dexeus S. Essure: a new device for hysteroscopic tubal sterilization in an outpatient setting. Fertil Steril 2004;82:196–9.
34. Gariepy AM, Crenin MD, Schwarz EB, et al. Reliability of laparoscopic compared with hysteroscopic sterilization at one year: a decision analysis. Obstet Gynecol 2011;118:273–9.
35. Panel P, Grosdemouge I. Predictive factors of Essure® implant placement failure: prospective, multicenter study of 495 patients. Fertil Steril 2010;93:29–34.
36. Leyser-Whalen O, Rouhani M, Rahman M, et al. Tubal risk markers for failure to place transcervical sterilization coils. Contraception 2012;85:384–8.
37. Cleary TP, Tepper NK, Cwiak C, et al. Pregnancies after hysteroscopic sterilization: a systematic review. Contraception 2013;87:539–48.
38. Rios-Castillo JE, Velasco E, Aronja-Berral JE, et al. Efficacy of Essure hysteroscopic sterilization—5 years follow up of 1200 women. Gynecol Endocrinol 2013;29:580–2.
39. Levie MD, Chudnoff SG. Prospective analysis of office-based hysteroscopic sterilization. J Minim Invasive Gynecol 2006;13:98–101.
40. Savage UK, Masters SJ, Smid MC, et al. Hysteroscopic sterilization in a large group practice. Obstet Gynecol 2009;114:1227–31.
41. Shavell VI, Abdallah ME, Diamond MP, et al. Post-Essure hysterosalpingography compliance in a clinic population. J Minim Invasive Gynecol 2008;15: 431–4.
42. Zurawin RK, Zurawin JL. Adverse events due to suspected nickel hypersensitivity in patients with Essure micro-inserts. J Minim Invasive Gynecol 2011; 18:475–82.

43. Hillis SD, Marchbanks PA, Tylor LR, et al, US Collaborative Review of Sterilization Working Group. Poststerilization regret: findings from the United States Collaborative Review of Sterilization. Obstet Gynecol 1999;93:889–95.
44. Chi IC, Jones BD. Incidence, risk factors, and prevention of poststerilization regret in women: an updated international review from an epidemiologic perspective. Obstet Gynecol Surv 1994;49:722–32.
45. Peterson HB, Xia Z, Hughes JM, et al. The risk for ectopic pregnancy after tubal sterilization. N Engl J Med 1997;336:762–7.
46. Trussell J. Contraceptive failure in the United States. Contraception 2011;83:397–404.
47. Giovannucci E, Tosteson TD, Speizer FE, et al. A long-term study of mortality rate in men who have undergone vasectomy. N Engl J Med 1992;326:1392.
48. Griffin T, Tooher R, Nowakowski K, et al. How little is enough? The evidence for post-vasectomy testing. J Urol 2005;147:29–36.
49. Grunert GM, Drake TS, Takaki NK. Microsurgical reanastamosis of the fallopian tube for reversal of sterilization. Obstet Gynecol 1981;58:148–51.
50. Dubuisson JB, Chapron C, Nos C, et al. Sterilization reversal: fertility results. Hum Reprod 1995;10:1145–51.
51. Deffieux X, Morin Surroca M, Faivre E, et al. Tubal anastomosis after tubal sterilization: a review. Arch Gynecol Obstet 2011;283:1149–58.
52. Gordts S, Campo R, Puttemans P, et al. Clinical factors determining pregnancy outcome after microsurgical tubal reanastamosis. Fertil Steril 2009;92:1198–202.
53. Rock JA, Guzick DS, Katz E, et al. Tubal anastomosis: pregnancy success following reversal of Falope ring or monopolar cautery sterilization. Fertil Steril 1987;48:13–7.
54. Fox M. Vasectomy reversal-microsurgery for best results. Br J Urol 1994;73:449–53.
55. Van Dongen J, Tekle FB, van Roijen JH. Pregnancy rate after vasectomy reversal in a contemporary series: influence of smoking, semen quality and post-surgical use of assisted reproductive techniques. BJU Int 2012;110:562–7.
56. Bolduc S, Fischer MA, Deceuninck G, et al. Factors predicting overall success: a review of 747 microsurgical vasovasostomies. Can Urol Assoc J 2007;1:388–94.
57. Trussell J, Lalla AM, Doan QV, et al. Cost-effectiveness of contraceptives in the United States. Contraception 2009;79:5–14.
58. Kraemer DF, Yen PY, Nichols M. An economic comparison of female sterilization of hysteroscopic tubal occlusion with laparoscopic bilateral tubal ligation. Contraception 2009;80:254–60.

Index

Note: Page numbers of article titles are in **boldface** type.

A

Abortion
  surgical
    IUD insertion after, **583–591** (*See also* Intrauterine device (IUD) insertion)
ACA. *See* Affordable Care Act (ACA)
Adolescent(s)
  cognitive development in, 632
  contraception for, **631–645**
    access to, 638–639
    barrier methods, 637
    CHC, 636–637
    contraceptive patch, 637
    contraceptive ring, 637
    copper IUD, 634–635
    discussion during reproductive health visit, 633
    ENG implant, 634
    introduction, 631–632
    IUDs
      special considerations for, 635
    LARC methods, 633
    LNG IUDs, 634
    options, 633–637
    POPs, 636
    postpregnancy insertion, 635
    progestin-only methods, 636
    successful programs for, 639
  high-risk behavior among, 632
  OTC access to OCs by, 623–624
  PID testing in, 635
  pregnancy in
    costs related to, 631–632
    prevalence of, 631–632
  reproductive health education for, 638
  STI testing in, 635
Adolescent health, 632
Adolescent reproductive health visit, 632–633
Affordable Care Act (ACA)
  contraceptive coverage and, **605–617**
    discussion, 613–614
  contraceptive coverage mandate, 607–614 (*See also* Contraceptive coverage mandate, of ACA)
  described, 605–607

Obstet Gynecol Clin N Am 42 (2015) 725–735
http://dx.doi.org/10.1016/S0889-8545(15)00102-3
0889-8545/15/$ – see front matter © 2015 Elsevier Inc. All rights reserved.

Affordable (*continued*)
   in family planning, 607
   implementation of
      challenges related to, 610–611
   legal challenges to, 609–610
   in Medicaid expansion, 607
   in preventive health care, 605–607
Antibiotic(s)
   before immediate IUD insertion after surgical abortion, 585
Antidiuretics
   for unscheduled bleeding associated with copper IUD, 596
Antifibrinolytic agents
   for unscheduled bleeding associated with copper IUD, 596
   for unscheduled bleeding associated with LNG IUD, 597
Antiprogestins
   for unscheduled bleeding associated with ENG implant, 600
   for unscheduled bleeding associated with LNG IUD, 598

B

Barrier methods
   in adolescent contraception, 637
Bleeding
   COCs and, 674–675
   unscheduled
      LARC–related
         therapeutic options for, **593–603** (*See also* Long-acting reversible contraception
            (LARC), unscheduled bleeding associated with, therapeutic options for)
BMI. *See* Body mass index (BMI)
Body mass index (BMI)
   contraceptive use related to, 649
   epidemiology of obesity and, 648–649
   sexual behavior related to, 649

C

Cesarean section
   sterilization with, 717
CHC. *See* Combined hormonal contraception (CHC)
COCs. *See* Combined oral contraceptives (COCs)
Combined hormonal contraception (CHC)
   for adolescents, 636–637
   bleeding profile with, 674–675
   efficacy of, 672–673
   initiation of
      examination and tests prior to, 665
   non-oral, 676–677
   progestogen in
      VTE risk related to, **683–698**
         background risks, 687–689
         introduction, 683–684

safety of, 673–674
Combined oral contraceptives (COCs), **669–681**
    bleeding profile with, 674–675
    efficacy of, 672–673
    extended and continuous
        development of, 671–672
    flexible and tailored regimens of, 676
    introduction, 669–670
    patient acceptability of, 675–676
    physiology of
        VTE related to, 686–687
    regimen types
        described, 670–671
    safety of, 673–674
    terminology related to, 670–671
    in treatment of menstrual symptoms, 675
Confidentiality
    during adolescent reproductive health visit, 633
Contraception. *See also specific methods*
    ACA and, 605–608
    for adolescents
        providing, **631–645** (*See also* Adolescent(s), contraception for)
    emergency, **699–712** (*See also* Emergency contraception (EC))
    hormonal
        without prescription
            women's interest in, 620–621
    initiation of
        after EC, 706
    long-acting reversible
        in decreasing unplanned pregnancy, **557–567** (*See* Long-acting reversible
            contraception (LARC))
    methods of (*See also specific methods*)
        initiation of, **659–667** (*See also* Contraceptive method initiation)
    in obese/overweight women, **647–657** (*See also* Obese/overweight women,
        contraceptive methods for)
    postpartum intrauterine
        immediate, **569–582** (*See also* Postpartum intrauterine contraception (PPIUC),
            immediate)
    weight effects of, 653–654
    in women of different BMIs, 649
Contraception CHOICE project, 639
Contraceptive CHOICE project, 563–564
Contraceptive coverage
    ACA on, **605–617** (*See also* Affordable Care Act (ACA))
Contraceptive coverage mandate
    of ACA, 607–608
        compliance with, 609
        discussion, 613–614
        legal challenges facing, 611–613
        limitations and inconsistencies with compliance to, 608–609
        Medicaid expansion and expanded contraceptive access, 608

Contraceptive (*continued*)
    no-cost contraceptive coverage expansion, 608
  implementation of
    status of
      progress and delays, 608–614
Contraceptive method initiation, **659–667**
  described, 660–663
  examination and tests prior to, 664–665
  follow-up care, 665
  introduction, 659–660
  postabortion, 664
  postpartum, 663
  in special circumstances, 663–664
Contraceptive patch
  in adolescents, 637
Contraceptive ring
  in adolescents, 637
  in obese/overweight women
    efficacy of, 651
Copper intrauterine device (Cu-IUD)
  in adolescents, 634–635
  described, 703
  in EU, 703–704
  mechanism of action of, 703
  safety of, 703
  side effects of, 703–704
  unscheduled bleeding associated with
    therapeutic options for, 594–596
Cu-IUD. *See* Copper intrauterine device (Cu-IUD)

D

Depot medroxyprogesterone acetate (DMPA)
  in adolescents, 636
  in obese/overweight women
    efficacy of, 650
DMPA. *See* Depot medroxyprogesterone acetate (DMPA)

E

EC. *See* Emergency contraception (EC)
Electrocoagulation
  laparoscopic
    in female sterilization, 715
Emergency contraception (EC), **699–712**
  copper IUD, 703–704
  increasing access to, 706–707
  introduction, 699–701
  LNG-containing EC pill, 705
  oral EC interactions with other medications, 706
  oral forms of, 704–705

pregnancy risk with, 701–703
    UPA in, 704
    when to start contraception after, 706
    Yuzpe method, 705–706
ENG implant. *See* Etonogestrel (ENG) implant
Estrogen
    for unscheduled bleeding associated with LNG IUD, 598
Etonogestrel (ENG) implant
    for adolescents, 634
    in obese/overweight women
        efficacy of, 650
    unscheduled bleeding associated with
        therapeutic options for, 598–601

F

Family planning
    ACA in, 607

G

Grandfathered plans
    contraceptive coverage mandate of ACA and, 608–609

H

Hysteroscopy
    microinserts placement via
        in transcervical sterilization, 718–719

I

Immediate intrauterine device (IUD) insertion
    after surgical abortion, **583–591** (*See also* Intrauterine device (IUD), immediate, after
        surgical abortion)
Injectable progestins
    in obese/overweight women
        efficacy of, 650
Insurance
    contraception for adolescents through, 638
Intrauterine device(s) (IUDs)
    in adolescents
        special considerations for, 635
    copper (*See* Copper intrauterine device (Cu-IUD))
    in obese/overweight women
        efficacy of, 649–650
Intrauterine device (IUD) insertion
    after first trimester surgical abortion, 585–586
    after second trimester surgical abortion, 586–587
    immediate
        after surgical abortion, **583–591**

Intrauterine (*continued*)
        background of, 583–584
        bleeding patterns, 587–588
        complications of, 588–589
        continuation and expulsion, 584
        follow-up care, 588
        patient experience with, 589
        preprocedure preparation, 584–585
        safety issues, 588–589
        ultrasound guidance in, 587
    initiation of
        examination and tests prior to, 664
IUDs. *See* Intrauterine device(s) (IUDs)

L

Laparoscopy
    in female sterilization, 714–717
        adverse effects of, 716
        comparison of techniques, 716
        electrocoagulation in, 715
        mechanical occlusion, 715–716
        tubal sterilization failure after, 716–717
LARC. *See* Long-acting reversible contraception (LARC)
Legal issues
    ACA–related, 609–610
Levonorgestrel (LNG)-containing emergency contraceptive pill, 705
Levonorgestrel (LNG) intrauterine device (IUD)
    for adolescents, 634
    unscheduled bleeding associated with
        therapeutic options for, 596–598
LNG IUD. *See* Levonorgestrel (LNG) intrauterine device (IUD)
Long-acting reversible contraception (LARC)
    for adolescents, 633
    in decreasing unplanned pregnancy, **557–567**
        barriers to use of, 559–562
            health care systems issues, 561–562
            providers issues, 561
            women's issues, 559–560
        increased use of, **557–567**
            in Colorado, 564
            Contraceptive CHOICE project, 563–564
            introduction, 557–558
            in Iowa, 564
            results of, 562–564
    OTC access to OCs effects on, 624
    unscheduled bleeding associated with
        therapeutic options for, **593–603**
            copper IUD, 594–596
            ENG implant, 598–601
            introduction, 593–594

LNG IUD, 596–598
vs. short-acting contraceptive methods
efficacy of, 558–559

M

Matrix metalloproteinase (MMP) inhibitors
for unscheduled bleeding associated with ENG implant, 600
MEC. *See* Medical Eligibility Criteria (MEC)
Mechanical occlusion
laparoscopic
in female sterilization, 715–716
Medicaid
ACA in expansion of, 607
contraception for adolescents through, 638–639
Medical Eligibility Criteria (MEC)
in contraceptive use among obese/overweight women, 652
Menstrual symptoms
treatment of
COCs in, 675
MMP inhibitors. *See* Matrix metalloproteinase (MMP) inhibitors

N

Non-oral combined hormonal contraception (CHC), 676–677
Nonsteroidal antiinflammatory drugs (NSAIDs)
for unscheduled bleeding
Cu-IUD–related, 595–596
ENG implant–related, 599–600
LNG IUD–related, 597
NSAIDs. *See* Nonsteroidal antiinflammatory drugs (NSAIDs)

O

Obese/overweight women
contraceptive efficacy in, 649–652
contraceptive methods for, **647–657**
efficacy of, 649–652
introduction, 647–648
pharmacodynamics of, 649–652
pharmacokinetics of, 649–652
risks related to, 652–653
Obesity
defined, 648
epidemiology of, 648–649
prevalence of, 647
OCs. *See* Oral contraceptives (OCs)
Open abdominal sterilization methods
female, 717
Opportunistic salpingectomy, 717–718
Oral contraceptives (OCs)
combined, **669–681** (*See also* Combined oral contraceptives (COCs))

Oral (*continued*)
   in obese/overweight women
      efficacy of, 650–651
   OTC access to, **619–629**
      adolescents use of, 623–624
      areas of concern related to, 623–625
      cost and insurance coverage issues, 623
      effectiveness of, 621–622
      introduction, 619–620
      lack of familiarity with POPs, 625
      lost opportunity to counsel about LARC methods related to, 624
      ongoing use
         evidence regarding, 622–623
      preventive screening related to, 624
      safety of, 621–622
      support among professional medical and nursing groups, 625–626
      women's interest in, 620–621
OTC access. *See* Over-the-counter (OTC) access
Over-the-counter (OTC) access
   to OCs, **619–629** (*See also* Oral contraceptives (OCs), OTC access to)
Overweight
   defined, 648

   P

Pelvic inflammatory disease (PID)
   testing for
      in adolescents, 635
Perforation
   IUD insertion after surgical abortion and, 588
PID. *see* Pelvic inflammatory disease (PID)
POPs. *See* Progestin-only pills (POPs)
Postabortion contraceptive method initiation, 664
Postpartum contraceptive method initiation, 663
Postpartum intrauterine contraception (PPIUC)
   described, 570
   immediate, **569–582**
      complications of, 579
      expulsion rate with, 578–579
      indications for, 570–571
      introduction, 569
      patient evaluation prior to, 579–581
      placement of, 571–578
PPIUC. *See* Postpartum intrauterine contraception (PPIUC)
Pregnancy
   EC and
      risks factors for, 701–703
   unplanned
      LARCS in decreasing, **557–567** (*See also* Long-acting reversible contraception
         (LARC), in decreasing unplanned pregnancy)
Preventive health care

ACA in, 605–607
Progestin(s)
    injectable
        in obese/overweight women
            efficacy of, 650
    third- and fourth-generation
        VTE risks related to
            contraceptive ring and patch, 692
            first pill scare, 691
            history of, 689–693
            prospective studies, 692–693
            second pill scare, 691–692
Progestin-only contraception
    in adolescents, 636
Progestin-only pills (POPs)
    for adolescents, 636
    lack of familiarity with
        OTC access to OCs and, 625
Progestogen(s)
    in CHC
        VTE risk related to, **683–698** (*See also* Combined hormonal contraception (CHC),
            progestogen in)
    types of, 684–686

S

Salpingectomy
    opportunistic, 717–718
School-based health centers
    contraception for adolescents at, 638
Selective progesterone receptor modulators
    for unscheduled bleeding associated with LNG IUD, 598
Sexual behavior
    discussion about
        during adolescent reproductive health visit, 633
    of women of different BMIs, 649
Sexually transmitted infections (STIs)
    discussion about
        during adolescent reproductive health visit, 633
    screening for
        before immediate IUD insertion after surgical abortion, 584–585
    testing for
        in adolescents, 635
Sterilization, **713–724**
    female
        after cesarean section, 717
        contraindications to, 720
        counseling related to, 719–720
        failure of, 720
        laparoscopy, 714–717 (*See also* Laparoscopy)
        open abdominal methods in, 717

Sterilization (*continued*)
    opportunistic salpingectomy, 717–718
    transcervical, 718–719
    tubal
      failure after laparoscopic sterilization, 716–717
  introduction, 713–714
  male, 720–721
    costs related to, 721
    sterilization reversal, 721
    vasectomy, 721
Sterilization reversal
  male, 721
STIs. *See* Sexually transmitted infections (STIs)
Surgical abortion
  first trimester
    IUD insertion after, 585–586
  immediate IUD insertion after, **583–591** (*See also* Intrauterine device (IUD) insertion,
    immediate, after surgical abortion)
  second trimester
    IUD insertion after, 586–587

T

Thromboembolism
  venous (*See* Venous thromboembolism (VTE))
Title X
  contraception for adolescents through, 638–639
Transcervical sterilization, 718–719
Transdermal patch
  in obese/overweight women
    efficacy of, 651–652
Tubal sterilization
  failure of
    after laparoscopic sterilization, 716–717

U

Ulipristal acetate (UPA)
  in EC, 704
Ultrasound
  in IUD placement after surgical abortion, 587
Unplanned pregnancy
  LARC in decreasing, **557–567** (*See also* Long-acting reversible contraception (LARC), in
    decreasing unplanned pregnancy)
  in women of different BMI groups, 648–649
UPA. *See* Ulipristal acetate (UPA)

V

Vaginal ring
  in adolescents, 637

in obese/overweight women
    efficacy of, 651
Vasectomy
  costs related to, 721
Venous thromboembolism (VTE)
  COCs physiology and, 686–687
  contraceptive use among obese/overweight women and, 652–653
  progestogen in CHC and, **683–698** (*See also* Combined hormonal contraception (CHC),
    progestogen in)
VTE. *See* Venous thromboembolism (VTE)

W

Weight
  contraceptive effects on, 653–654

Y

Yuzpe method
  in EC, 705–706

United States Postal Service

Statement of Ownership, Management, and Circulation
(All Periodicals Publications Except Requester Publications)

1. Publication Title
Obstetrics and Gynecology Clinics of North America

2. Publication Number
0 0 0 - 2 7 7 6

3. Filing Date
9/18/15

4. Issue Frequency
Mar, Jun, Sep, Dec

5. Number of Issues Published Annually
4

6. Annual Subscription Price
$310.00

7. Complete Mailing Address of Known Office of Publication *(Not printer) (Street, city, county, state, and ZIP+4®)*
Elsevier Inc.
360 Park Avenue South
New York, NY 10010-1710

Contact Person
Stephen R. Bushing

Telephone *(Include area code)*
215-239-3688

8. Complete Mailing Address of Headquarters or General Business Office of Publisher *(Not printer)*
Elsevier Inc., 360 Park Avenue South, New York, NY 10010-1710

9. Full Names and Complete Mailing Addresses of Publisher, Editor, and Managing Editor *(Do not leave blank)*

Publisher *(Name and complete mailing address)*
Linda Belfus, Elsevier Inc., 1600 John F. Kennedy Blvd., Suite 1800, Philadelphia, PA 19103

Editor *(Name and complete mailing address)*
Kerry Holland, Elsevier Inc., 1600 John F. Kennedy Blvd., Suite 1800, Philadelphia, PA 19103-2899

Managing Editor *(Name and complete mailing address)*
Adrianne Brigido, Elsevier Inc., 1600 John F. Kennedy Blvd., Suite 1800, Philadelphia, PA 19103-2899

10. Owner *(Do not leave blank. If the publication is owned by a corporation, give the name and address of the corporation immediately followed by the names and addresses of all stockholders owning or holding 1 percent or more of the total amount of stock. If not owned by a corporation, give the names and addresses of the individual owners. If owned by a partnership or other unincorporated firm, give its name and address as well as those of each individual owner. If the publication is published by a nonprofit organization, give its name and address.)*

Full Name	Complete Mailing Address
Wholly owned subsidiary of	1600 John F. Kennedy Blvd., Ste. 1800
Reed/Elsevier, US holdings	Philadelphia, PA 19103-2899

11. Known Bondholders, Mortgagees, and Other Security Holders Owning or Holding 1 Percent or More of Total Amount of Bonds, Mortgages, or Other Securities. If none, check box ☐ None

Full Name	Complete Mailing Address
N/A	

12. Tax Status *(For completion by nonprofit organizations authorized to mail at nonprofit rates) (Check one)*
The purpose, function, and nonprofit status of this organization and the exempt status for federal income tax purposes:
☐ Has Not Changed During Preceding 12 Months
☐ Has Changed During Preceding 12 Months *(Publisher must submit explanation of change with this statement)*

13. Publication Title
Obstetrics and Gynecology Clinics of North America

14. Issue Date for Circulation Data Below
September 2015

15. Extent and Nature of Circulation			Average No. Copies Each Issue During Preceding 12 Months	No. Copies of Single Issue Published Nearest to Filing Date
a. Total Number of Copies *(Net press run)*			729	562
b. Legitimate Paid and Or Requested Distribution (By Mail and Outside the Mail)	(1)	Mailed Outside County Paid/Requested Mail Subscriptions stated on PS Form 3541. *(Include paid distribution above nominal rate, advertiser's proof copies and exchange copies)*	227	117
	(2)	Mailed In-County Paid/Requested Mail Subscriptions stated on PS Form 3541. *(Include paid distribution above nominal rate, advertiser's proof copies and exchange copies)*		
	(3)	Paid Distribution Outside the Mails Including Sales Through Dealers And Carriers, Street Vendors, Counter Sales, and Other Paid Distribution Outside USPS®	218	265
	(4)	Paid Distribution by Other Classes of Mail Through the USPS (e.g. First-Class Mail®)		
c. Total Paid and or Requested Circulation *(Sum of 15b (1), (2), (3), and (4))*			445	382
d. Free or Nominal Rate Distribution (By Mail and Outside the Mail)	(1)	Free or Nominal Rate Outside-County Copies included on PS Form 3541	46	44
	(2)	Free or Nominal Rate In-County Copies included on PS Form 3541		
	(3)	Free or Nominal Rate Copies mailed at Other classes Through the USPS (e.g. First-Class Mail®)		
	(4)	Free or Nominal Rate Distribution Outside the Mail *(Carriers or Other means)*		
e. Total Nonrequested Distribution *(Sum of 15d (1), (2), (3) and (4))*			46	44
f. Total Distribution *(Sum of 15c and 15e)*			491	426
g. Copies not Distributed *(See instructions to publishers #4 (page #3))*			238	136
h. Total *(Sum of 15f and g)*			729	562
i. Percent Paid and/or Requested Circulation *(15c divided by 15f times 100)*			90.63%	89.67%

* If you are claiming electronic copies go to line 16 on page 3. If you are not claiming Electronic copies, skip to line 17 on page 3.

16. Electronic Copy Circulation	Average No. Copies Each Issue During Preceding 12 Months	No. Copies of Single Issue Published Nearest to Filing Date
a. Paid Electronic Copies		
b. Total paid Print Copies *(Line 15c)* + Paid Electronic copies *(Line 16a)*		
c. Total Print Distribution *(Line 15f)* + Paid Electronic Copies *(Line 16a)*		
d. Percent Paid (Both Print & Electronic copies) *(16b divided by 16c X 100)*		

☐ I certify that 50% of all my distributed copies (electronic and print) are paid above a nominal price

17. Publication of Statement of Ownership
If the publication is a general publication, publication of this statement is required. Will be printed in the ___December 2015___ issue of this publication.

18. Signature and Title of Editor, Publisher, Business Manager, or Owner

Stephen R. Bushing

Date
September 18, 2015

Stephen R. Bushing – Inventory Distribution Coordinator

I certify that all information furnished on this form is true and complete. I understand that anyone who furnishes false or misleading information on this form or who omits material or information requested on the form may be subject to criminal sanctions (including fines and imprisonment) and/or civil sanctions (including civil penalties).

PS Form **3526**, July 2014 (Page 1 of 3 [Instructions Page 3]) PSN 7530-01-000-9931 **PRIVACY NOTICE:** See our Privacy policy in www.usps.com

PS Form 3526, July 2014 (Page 3 of 3)

Moving?

Make sure your subscription moves with you!

To notify us of your new address, find your **Clinics Account Number** (located on your mailing label above your name), and contact customer service at:

Email: journalscustomerservice-usa@elsevier.com

800-654-2452 (subscribers in the U.S. & Canada)
314-447-8871 (subscribers outside of the U.S. & Canada)

Fax number: 314-447-8029

Elsevier Health Sciences Division
Subscription Customer Service
3251 Riverport Lane
Maryland Heights, MO 63043

*To ensure uninterrupted delivery of your subscription, please notify us at least 4 weeks in advance of move.

Printed and bound by CPI Group (UK) Ltd, Croydon, CR0 4YY

03/10/2024

01040492-0018